THE
NATURAL
SOAP
BOOK

MAKING HERBAL AND
VEGETABLE-BASED SOAPS

SUSAN MILLER CAVITCH

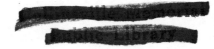

STOREY BOOKS

Schoolhouse Road
Pownal, Vermont 05261

The mission of Storey Communications is to serve our customers by publishing practical information that encourages personal independence in harmony with the environment.

Edited by Deborah L. Balmuth
Cover, text design, and production by Carol J. Jessop, Black Trout Design
Cover and text illustrations ©John Nelson/Represented by Irmeli Holmberg
Line drawings by Brigita Fuhrmann
Indexed by Northwind Editorial Services

Printed in the United States by R.R. Donnelley
10   9   8   7

Library of Congress Cataloging-in-Publication Data

Cavitch, Susan Miller, 1959–
        The natural soap book : making herbal and vegetable-based soaps/ Susan Miller
   Cavitch.
             p.   cm.

        Includes bibliographical references (p.   ) and index.
        ISBN 0-88266-888-9 (pbk.)
        1. Soap. I. Title.
   TP991.C39   1995
   668'.12—dc20   95-6061
                                                                                            CIP

TABLE OF CONTENTS

PART ONE: Understanding the Basics

PART TWO: The Ingredients

PART THREE: Making Soap

PART FOUR: Beyond the Basics

"Leave a little to nature: she understands her business better than we do."
Montaigne, *Essays*, A.D. 1595

For Matt,
and for Peter, Jenny, Adam, and Mary,
my connection to,
and my greatest gifts from,
the Lord and His Gospel.

Matt, my husband, my buddy, my editor, and my favorite author.
You saw this book before I did, and you shared it with me, as we've shared so
much else. You've taught me and our children how to press forward,
past distraction and ill winds.

Peter, who just as I'm fading, pops into my workroom with an offer to help.
You are a good worker with a kind heart, and I appreciate all that you've
done for me.

Jenny, who is interested in everything and everyone, and whose enthusiasm
is infectious. You keep my wonder cells alive.

Adam, my farmer, who instinctively appreciates nature and the need to
conserve our resources. Your gentle way will make a difference.

Mary, my comic relief, whose hugs and lusty laughter keep things
in perspective.

ACKNOWLEDGMENTS

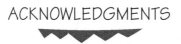

I'd like to acknowledge several people who have been of great help to me without even knowing it.

Macky Miller, my mother, who has always been there for me. Your love and nerve spread my early soaps across state lines. You have given my products as gifts to the same people year after year, and, though I know you like my soaps and feel good about giving them, I know better why you've done it.

Harris Miller, my father, a great listener, who lets me bounce ideas and troubles off of him, soapwise and otherwise. You spent countless hours prodding me toward computer literacy — long-distance, often after midnight, and always with patience and humor.

Steve Miller, my brother, who as a feisty five-year-old could do no wrong by me — whose undisciplined honesty developed over time into mature truthfulness. The little brother you nurtured becomes the adult who nurtures you right back. You listened and responded to talk of juniper berry meal and shea butter when you had other things on your mind, and you always bothered to ask for progress reports. Thank you.

Betsy Cohen, my sister, for her conditional seal of approval. When she began calling for refills, I knew I was on the right track. Perhaps no two people share as much history in common as two sisters who grew up just a couple of years apart. You and Steve could always make me laugh, and I'm grateful for all of the laughter.

Sylvia Fish, my grandmother, who has been a second mother to me. You have fed a constant supply of love and fun into my life.

Heidi Hurwitz, my friend and confidante, who instinctively understands. You taught me through example to put myself on the line, as is, with no pretention. You love completely and honestly, because you take nothing for granted and deeply appreciate all of the gifts. Thank you for thinking creatively for me when I ran low.

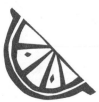

Gertrude LeVine, my great-aunt, who has always shared with me, and I with her, as if there were no age difference.

Alfred Weller, my great-uncle, who took me under his wing throughout my college days and never pushed me out of the nest. I still call long-distance the only pediatrician I thoroughly trust.

Danny Klein, my uncle, who gives wholeheartedly and lightens things up. Your enthusiasm inspires the rest of us to take time to play.

Linda Griffith, my cousin, who surrounds herself with color and inspires so many of us to see the art in all things. You have always recognized your knowledge and talents as gifts, passing them along freely to others. This example encourages the rest of us to be forthright and generous.

Pernille Våge, a friend brought to me from across the ocean in a most unlikely way. Long before you offered me your creative efforts, I considered you a gift. Thank you for lasting designs and lasting impressions.

Urania Erskine, my friend, whose faith and humility allow great works to flow through her. No nonsense and good humor are indeed compatible, for they are the best of companions within you. I'm grateful for the fires you've started beneath me.

Sally Whipple, my friend, the cookie lady. Grandma babysits in her eighties and affects all of her children with her pure faith. Your example reminds us all to take the time to walk the aisles slowly, to chat over a cup of tea with a friend, and to talk to our photographs.

Deborah Balmuth, my editor at Storey Communications, who made this a better book. Though I'm in Tennessee, and Deborah is in Vermont, and though we were complete strangers up until recently, I have been enriched by the short time we've worked as a team. Thank you for your professionally persistent, yet gentle, criticism.

The chemist, who shall remain nameless, who was helpful and friendly from day one — whose New Jersey accent and New Jersey wit kept me laughing, in spite of my failures.

And a few others I miss daily, but feel nearby: Mary and Harry Weller, my great-grandparents, who showed me all I needed to know about appreciating your eternal mates; Maurice and Freida Miller, my grandparents, who took the time to fuss over us, and whose open-door policy offered me one of my quietest places; my grandfather, Albert Fish, a real gentleman, who brought out the best in people and didn't judge the least; and Marie and Jean Berthelot, who adopted me as their own and taught me to work hard, and who put German and French lullabies into my head.

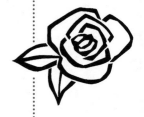

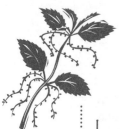

PREFACE

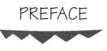

In August 1990, I visited a tourist trap in Arkansas, where I watched a middle-aged woman dressed in a pioneer costume make soap in an iron kettle over a hole in the ground. For three dollars, I purchased a bar of her soap. The bar was 12 hours old, wet and mushy. She slid it into a plastic baggy and told me to let it sit out for a few days. "It's better that way." This was my introduction to soapmaking. I was enthralled.

Within one week the soap had shrivelled and spotted with little brown circles. I telephoned the woman in the costume and she reassured me, "Oh honey, that's fine. That's the way it's supposed to be."

It has taken me three years to know what I know now. Though I am far from the greatest expert on soapmaking, I have learned that the production of soap does not have to be completed by the purchaser. I have also learned that vegetable soaps do not have to be soft, that there is more than one right temperature for soapmaking, that preservatives do not have to be seven-syllable synthetics, and that a soapmaker does not have to be a chemist to understand enough to figure out solutions. It has taken me three years to sort out fact from fiction when it comes to soapmakers and their theories of soapmaking. I write this book so that the next hopeful soapmaker can save a little time.

Along the way, I have spoken with many soapmakers, several chemists, and dozens of suppliers. I have read books on both soapmaking and chemistry, and have been confused and frustrated by the inconsistencies among the many things I've heard or read. Most people have been refreshingly eager to help me understand soapmaking, but some people have not, treating their knowledge as a trade secret. Protecting one's business or occupation is undeniably legitimate, but it still irks me. I resolved early on in my soapmaking experiences that I would share my knowledge if I ever got any. This book is dedicated to that resolution.

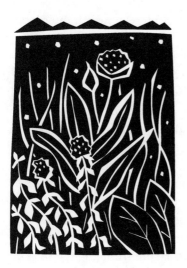

Understanding

The

Basics

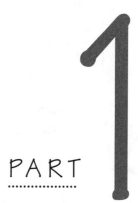

PART

INTRODUCTION

$\mathcal{S}$oap can be made from fats and oils, sodium hydroxide, and water. Soapmaking can be as simple as dissolving sodium hydroxide in water, melting fats together, adding the sodium hydroxide solution (lye) to the melted fats, and stirring. It can get more complicated, but it needn't. This book starts at the beginning, assuming the reader knows nothing about soapmaking. Chemistry is discussed, but in digestible portions and only enough to get a good working feel for the observable process. I survived high school chemistry only with the help of a motivated friend. I am well aware that those kinds of friends and that kind of motivation are not so common anymore for me and my post-teenage readers. Accordingly, this book has been written sympathetically, for the reader who does not have an interpreter. The chapters are arranged to take you step-by-step up to, through, and beyond the soapmaking process.

Part One introduces you to six different ways of classifying soaps. Part Two describes, in detail, the many soapmaking ingredients. Part Three explains how to make soap, from choosing the equipment to cutting and trimming the final bars.

In Part Four, I take you "Beyond the Basics," to encourage creativity in wrapping and presenting your soaps. I also provide a more detailed discussion of the chemistry of soapmaking, reminding the reader to rejoice that soapmaking is more art than science.

Scattered throughout this book, you will find the stories of a handful of commercially successful American soapmakers who share their experience and trace their journeys through soapmaking.

The appendices include a list of suppliers from whom you can buy soapmaking ingredients, a glossary, and a list of related reading material.

WHAT IS SOAP?

Chemically — and I'll explain this in detail later — soap is a salt. An acid and a base react with one another and neutralize into the salt (or soap). This process is called *saponification;* as the acid and the base come into contact with one another and react, the solution is saponifying — making soap. There are many forms of acids and bases and many different ways of making soap. One method relies upon sodium hydroxide for the base, another sodium carbonate, and yet another potassium hydroxide. One method uses fats and oils for the acid, another just the pure fatty acids already split from the fat. One method releases glycerin, another doesn't. One involves boiling the soap in commercial kettles that hold several hundred thousand pounds, another is made in a small pan on your kitchen counter.

All of these methods produce soap, but most are beyond the scope of this book and the interest of humankind. Home-made bars are manufactured with fats and oils (the acid), sodium hydroxide (the base), and water (the solvent which dissolves the base). Making soap with easily accessible materials, without complex chemical additives, and using only the heat of the reaction (no external heat), is called the *cold-process method.* This book is about making soap most simply — using fats and oils, sodium hydroxide, and the cold-process method.

All-Vegetable Soaps

The same cold-process method used to make animal-based (tallow or lard) soaps can be used to make all-vegetable soaps. Though some soapmaking manuals include vegetable formulas, they fail to explain that making vegetable soaps requires some adjustments.

While the basic method remains the same, slight variations in the temperament of each vegetable oil call for special attention. Vegetable oils cannot tolerate the high temperatures that animal tallow can withstand, require different amounts of sodium hydroxide, can take longer to saponify (make soap), require different preservatives, and cure differently as soaps. Formulas incorporating a high percentage of beef tallow can be made at higher temperatures. When vegetable soaps are made at high temperatures, the mixture curdles more easily, produces a grainier soap, and has a tough time incorporating the essential oils.

The soapmaker who is interested in researching tallow/lard-based soaps has plenty of existing material to read; this book emphasizes vegetable-based soaps and their individual characteristics and complexities.

Once you understand basic soapmaking chemistry, and which laws must be followed and which ones can be defied, then you can play with the formulas. There is no one right way to make soap, but I will guide you to successful soapmaking.

HOW DOES SOAP CLEAN?

Before focusing too narrowly on the details of soapmaking, it is worth pausing for a moment to understand how soap works. To clean skin or fabric, something must make the surface wet and attract the dirt away. Soap does both.

THE DISCOVERY OF SOAP

The story told in 1,000 B.C. Rome, about the discovery of soap on Sapo Hill, has been repeated so often that mythical elements have taken on factual proportions.

The story tells of women rinsing clothes in the river at the base of a hill, below a higher elevation where animal sacrifice had taken place. They noticed the clothes coming clean as they came in contact with the soapy clay oozing down the hill and into the water. They later discovered that this cleansing substance was formed when the rendered animal fat soaked down through the wood ashes and into the clay soil.

Ironically, water alone does not wet well. Water molecules are closely bonded and resist being broken apart. They bead up on the surface and do not spread out easily. Soap acts as a *surfactant,* or a surface active agent, which means that it helps the water to soak in rather than form tight droplets. Soap molecules have heads which attract water, and tails which repel it. When mixed with water, these soap molecules push their hydrophobic tails up through the surface of the water, to get as far away as possible. All of these tails poking through the top layer break up the surface tension of the water and cause it to spread out and wet more thoroughly.

Soap removes dirt and grease in two stages. First, it attaches itself to the dirt, and then it suspends the dirt in lather until a rinse carries them both away. More specifically, a soap molecule is a chain of atoms — including carbon, hydrogen, and oxygen — arranged with a distinct head and tail. The head is attracted to water, the tail to dirt. The soap molecule cleans by embedding its tail into the dirt and dislodging it as its head pulls toward the water. The soap then holds the dirt in suspension until it's rinsed away.

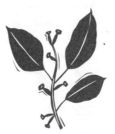

CHAPTER 1
The Kinds of Soap

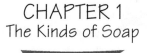

Not so long ago, a sliver of soap made from the leftover drippings of a month of meals was a treasure. It was highly caustic, and in great demand. These lard bars were a blessing to those who lived during the 17th and 18th centuries, but they were crude in comparison to what we have available to us today.

Our choices are many — maybe too many — and our work is cut out for us if we insist upon knowing exactly what we're using on our skin. For years before I became a soapmaker, I was thrilled by a display of elegantly wrapped bars, one the color of avocados, another with the scent of fresh gardenias, all polished smooth as gems and arranged on the shelves like pieces of crystal. The classical music playing in the background was a sure sign of the soap's purity. Today I'm not so easily wowed.

The stores are filled with all kinds of soaps. We may want liquid soap at the kitchen sink and solid bars in the bathtub. Many soaps are made with animal fats, and some are made with only vegetable oils. Most bars are manufactured industrially, while some are made in someone's kitchen. Some of the unusual shapes we see are milled through expensive machinery. Some soaps are actually detergents. Occasionally, we can find a bar that was manufactured without any synthetic chemicals at all. Let's take a closer look at the pros and cons of the soaps from which we can choose.

LIQUID SOAPS VERSUS BAR SOAPS

Liquid soaps offer convenience, cleanliness, and efficiency. They require very little effort to produce a lather, minimize person-to-person contact, and keep waste down.

Public restrooms usually offer liquid soap dispensers in place of bar soap to avoid messy counters, sloppy soap dishes, and the spread of germs. Surgeons use liquid soap with germicides for hospital scrubs, and many families place decorator dispensers by bathroom and kitchen sinks to keep things neat.

There is a price for this convenience, however. Many more chemicals are used to manufacture liquid soap than are necessary to manufacture a bar of hard soap. Certain synthetic chemicals are added to give the soap just the right consistency, so it doesn't clog the dispenser. Others are used to assure enough of a lather for the average squirt of soap. Liquid soaps feel smooth, smell fresh, and minimize cleanup, but their chemical makeup should be considered carefully.

Hard bars often contain as many chemicals as liquid soap, but they don't have to. This book is about hard soaps that are free of synthetic chemicals.

ANIMAL SOAPS VERSUS VEGETABLE SOAPS

Soaps made with animal fat contain tallow or lard, while vegetable-based soaps are made with just vegetable oils. More tallow is used in soapmaking than any other fat, but today you can find soap made with almost any oil imaginable. Some of us have a strong preference for either animal or vegetable soaps; others never give it a thought.

Tallow comes from the solid fat around the kidneys and loins of cattle, sheep, and horses. Lard is the fat rendered from the tissue of pigs. Both have been used for centuries in soapmaking, though increased access to coconut, olive, palm, and other fine vegetable oils has led soapmakers to experiment with all sorts of combinations. One oil may offer a wonderful lather, but have a drying effect when used in excess. Another oil may work up a weak lather, but cure into a very hard bar of soap. Yet another oil may make a softer bar, but clean well.

Just one fat or oil on its own is not likely to serve your needs; a carefully calculated combination of fats and oils yields a superior bar of soap.

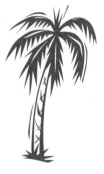

Availability and Cost of Ingredients

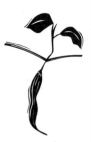

Whether you're looking for tallow, olive oil, or babassu oil, with enough persistence you'll find a supplier. You probably can find a meat processing plant within a drive of your home that will package the suet (see page 28) for you at no cost or a small per-pound price. Many fat and oil manufacturers or distributors carry pre-rendered tallow and lard in 50-pound buckets, saving the soapmaker the messy chore of rendering the suet into a usable liquid. This is more expensive, but quite a convenience. Rendering suet at home is a messy, time-consuming process.

Vegetable fats and oils may be more costly than tallow or lard, but their quality affords a superior skin-care product. And, purchasing vegetable oils in bulk 55-gallon drums, or even 50-pound buckets, makes them more affordable than the small decorator bottles of oil found at the supermarket. Oils that are commonly used in many industries, such as olive, are easier to find and less expensive to purchase than the more obscure oils.

Restaurant supply houses carry many of the edible oils in quantity. Bakeries and their suppliers used palm oil for years before health concerns about the oil's highly saturated makeup caused them to cut back. Palm oil is now sold mostly by the tank-car to fat and oil companies that break it down into drums and pails and sell directly to soapmakers or distributors. Call your local Italian restaurants and ask who supplies their olive oil. Call Oriental restaurants about peanut oil. Coconut oil is used by businesses selling popcorn, but avoid the orange variety, which is discolored with beta-carotene. Also avoid the expensive little 12-ounce jars of coconut oil.

Soapmakers will quickly go through the 50-pound pails or boxes sold by edible oil manufacturers and their distributors. Some oils — like jojoba, sweet almond, and castor — are far more expensive to buy in small quantity than in bulk, but 32-ounce bottles and gallons are available if you cannot use drums. If you prefer vegetable soaps to tallow soaps, it's worth taking the time to track down the desired oils in the quantities you can use. Even the more obscure varieties are available, one way or another. Keep calling around — you'll have no problem finding a company to satisfy your particular soapmaking needs (see *Suppliers* listed in the appendices, page 157).

Effect on Skin

Much controversy surrounds the use of tallow (or its synthetic equivalents) in skin-care products, especially soap. Some argue that it has cleaned many generations of people without harm. Others point to tallow as just one of many impurities unknowingly slathered onto our faces. Some experts view it in perspective: For thousands of years tallow was a godsend, enabling less well-supplied generations to maintain certain sanitary levels. Now, however, we have healthier alternatives. Tallow is highly saturated and thought to clog pores, causing blackheads. It is also known to cause eczema in more sensitive individuals. Moreover, some people have ethical objections to tallow because it is not derived from live animals.

Our skin works as hard as the rest of our organs, continually ridding the body of impurities and absorbing light and moisture. Skin readily accepts a variety of water and oil-soluble materials through the pores. Since both the good and the bad enter readily, we must consider carefully which products to use. Our skin acts as a protective barrier, even repairing itself from injury, but each toxic exposure damages this barrier and inhibits the skin's ability to function.

The general health of skin is related directly to its moisture content — how much water it's able to retain. As healthy skin "cleans house" under normal conditions, it can retain moisture; but heat, cold, pollution, ultraviolet rays, synthetic cosmetics, and an over-processed, less nutritious diet push our skin past its limits. It just can't keep up. If we don't conserve our skin's moisture content, the imbalance leads to dry skin and a less efficient system.

We need skin-care products that help the skin to balance its loss and absorption of moisture, while also nourishing the body with vitamins. Such products create a breathable barrier for the skin, attracting and allowing in a fresh supply of moisture while preventing the evaporation of internal moisture.

Tallow and lard can clog up the skin's breathing system. In contrast, a thin layer of certain vegetable oils will keep internal moisture from evaporating too quickly, while still allowing the skin to release waste and absorb a fresh supply of external moisture. Choose oils for soapmaking with an understanding of

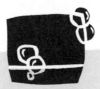

A SOAPMAKER'S STORY

Sandie Ledray and Mary McIsaac/Brookside Soap Company

The women of Brookside Soap Company, Sandie Ledray and Mary McIsaac, create herbal body-care products which "maximize and celebrate the power and richness of the plant kingdom, without exploiting people or the environment." Toward this goal, Brookside products contain no colorants, no synthetic ingredients, and nothing of animal origin. Their packaging is minimal and recyclable. The ink used on their soap wrappers is soy-based, and the glue to seal them is vegetable-based. The herbs used in their products are organically grown. The combinations range from Rosemary & Lavender Soap, with apricot kernel oil and chamomile flowers for all skin types, to Avocado and Calendula Soap with shea butter, oils of avocado, calendula, and apricot kernel, marshmallow root, and the essential oils of ylang-ylang, clove, and sage for normal to dry skin, and Cinnamon Hand Scrub with ground corn and cinnamon for gardeners, cooks, potters, and painters.

"Soapmaking found its way into my life rather by accident," says Sandie. When she ran out of funds while renovating her house, Sandie turned to her own resourcefulness, and began gardening, fishing — and making her own soap. Her very first batch turned out beautifully, and before long she was receiving visitors with empty buckets and dirty clothes. "As friends would walk out my door carrying a bucket of laundry soap, they would often suggest that I consider selling my great soap," says Sandie. It got to the point where she would have no peace until she began to heed her friends' requests. "My laundry soap turned into a bath bar soap," says Sandie, "which turned into an all-vegetable bath bar soap, which eventually turned into an organic, herbal bath bar soap line."

Sandie didn't have any soapmaker friends to help her perfect her product. "The high quality of our soap comes from years of trial and lots of error," says Sandie. "I have a record of every batch of soap that I have ever made, including its success or failure. Failure is good — you learn a tremendous amount about the materials and the chemistry from the failures!"

Today, Brookside Soaps are produced in 4,500 square feet of manufacturing space in a small business park in Seattle, Washington. They make 450-pound batches of cold-process soap, which is wire-cut by hand, and produce 28 different bar soaps, including eight Brookside Soaps and many private labels.

this function in mind. Some emollient oils that absorb moisture well are olive oil, castor oil, avocado oil, jojoba oil, and sweet almond oil.

Availability and Cost

All-vegetable soaps are not as scarce as they used to be, but tallow-based and synthetically manufactured soaps are still the norm. Because the cost of fine-quality vegetable oils is higher than that of tallow, most soapmaking companies find all-vegetable bars prohibitively expensive to produce. Tallow is relatively inexpensive and less temperamental during the soapmaking process, so it is the fat of choice for many soap manufacturers. However, as demand grows for soaps with fewer chemicals, no animal products, and skin-friendly vegetable oils, some companies are trying vegetable soaps and discovering that the manufacturing process is quite workable.

Still, tallow soaps and soaps made with synthetics comprise most of the products found in drugstores, supermarkets, and boutiques. To find all-vegetable soaps look for health food stores, mail-order businesses, and herbal gift shops. A pure vegetable-soap bar is usually more costly, though many tallow and synthetic soaps with fancy packaging carry similar price tags. When you buy soap, be sure that you are paying mostly for soap ingredients, not for packaging and presentation.

Texture and Lather

Many factors determine a soap's ability to lather and to remain firm throughout use. These qualities are related directly to which oils or fats were used in the soapmaking process. The more saturated a fat, the less soluble its soap will be in water, which also means that its lather will be weak, though longer lasting. Beef tallow and pork lard produce bars with weak lathers, while coconut oil, with its high proportion of lauric acid, offers a full lather, even in seawater. Olive, peanut, and soybean oils lather somewhat, but produce a superior lather only in combination with coconut oil. Companies producing tallow-based soaps usually add 20 percent coconut oil to achieve a satisfactory lather.

It is often claimed that tallow yields a much harder soap than a vegetable oil could and that harder soaps are longer-lasting and more economical. Tallow does make a very firm product, but vegetable oils can do the same. The combination of oils is key to making a hard vegetable soap. The right proportions of selected oils can produce a very hard bar — one that does not melt in the soap dish and lasts as long as a tallow soap. A variety of vegetable oils, combined with carefully calculated percentages of coconut and palm oils, produces a desirable texture and a long-lasting soap.

Again, keep in mind that industrially prepared soap is very different from cold-process soaps made by hand, without synthetics. The industrial soaps often rely upon synthetics to achieve physical characteristics like lather and texture. Most cold-processed soapmakers depend only upon oils and soapmaking techniques to achieve a desired result.

Scent

Both tallow soaps and vegetable-based soaps can be scented with pure essential oils and fragrance oils. The scent is more stable in vegetable-based soaps, however, because the natural odor of vegetable oils is less overpowering than the natural odor of tallow and lard. While vegetable oils are either odorless or very mild, animal fats may smell fatty and somewhat like their meat. In soap form, the vegetable oils remain odorless or mildly complementary of the pure essential or fragrance oils used, while the tallow or lard soaps may smell increasingly fatty, and overpower the pure essential or fragrance oils.

Choice is Personal

No one oil or fat is the clear-cut first choice for soapmaking. Each one has its own set of characteristics that contributes positively and negatively to the soap made from it. Animal-based soaps are not always inferior, and vegetable-based soaps are not always better. The most cooperative oil or fat must be selected for each characteristic desired in a soap. It is a combination of oils and fats that will yield the bar which satisfies the most needs. My preference for vegetable soaps is partly a personal philosophical choice.

HOMEMADE SOAPS VERSUS STORE-BOUGHT SOAPS

Though many areas of the cosmetic industry are bound by ingredient disclosure laws, an exception permits soap manufacturers to reveal only what they choose to reveal about their soaps. This makes it very difficult for consumers to know what they're using on their skin. Cottage industry and home manufacturing operations hardly have a monopoly on safe, effective skin-care products; larger companies often employ chemists and quality-control people to continually monitor their products for purity. However, "big business" historically has been pressured by the need to surpass the last quarter's profits, which often leads to compromising a soap's purity to achieve an impressive balance sheet. Though some companies offer superior products, we unfortunately cannot count on the large soap-producing industry to provide the purity and the quality we think we're purchasing.

Cottage industry affords consumers the opportunity to speak directly with the soapmaker, allowing for a more personal exchange, and, perhaps, a more reliable assessment of the integrity of their product. However, even this route leaves room for doubt. The only way to be sure of what goes into your soap is to make it yourself.

Homemade soap has no limits other than the energy and the imagination of the soapmaker. When you make your own soap you can use only the oils and the special ingredients individually suited to your skin-care needs. You don't have to wonder what has been added, skimped on, or left out, because you've seen for yourself what's gone into it.

MILLED SOAPS VERSUS HAND-CUT SOAPS

Milled soaps are made by machines that press freshly made soap between sets of rollers to flatten it paper thin and prepare it to be shredded. Once shredded, the soap flakes are ground through the rollers again and again, squeezing and mixing them together. The mixture then goes through extrusion machinery, that squeezes out a long bar of tightly compacted soap flakes, and cuts it into smaller bars. The flakes are no longer distinguishable within these dense bars of milled soap. The continuous compression creates a very hard soap and a polished appearance, while the very thin flakes increase the soap's lathering quality.

These soaps are truly beautiful, but we, as consumers, must remember to focus on content. Milled soaps rarely are made without tallow and many synthetic chemicals. A cold-processed vegetable soap with lots of unsaturated olive oil, no additives, and an excess of glycerin would stick to the rollers and extrude poorly. The milling industry typically adds a variety of synthetic chemicals to transform soap from its more natural state, and give it enough plasticity to withstand the milling process.

SHARING THE SECRETS OF SOAPMAKING

The only way to advance soapmaking research is for the soapmaker and the chemist to combine efforts, but we're as secretive today as people were in the 1700s, when they had even less information to share. In 1769, the Academy of Marseilles offered a prize for the research paper revealing the best method for making soap. There were no responses for five years. Finally, a man who later admitted to knowing nothing about soapmaking submitted a paper describing a particular method. It turned out he had acquired the information confidentially from a soapmaker friend.

Hand-cut bars are not always cold-process soaps made without additives, but they often are. Cottage industries usually make soap simply, with only fats, oils, sodium hydroxide, natural emollients, water, and essential oils. With the cold-process method, soap retains the natural glycerin created during the saponification process, and no chemicals are used to alter the natural reactions. With nothing added and nothing taken away, the final product is soap and not a laboratory imitation. Hand-cut bars are never perfectly squared or rounded; they appear rather crude when compared to a perfectly symmetrical, beautifully polished bar of milled soap. They also are far more prone to having excess fat or lye, since the cold-process method does not allow for adjustments once the reaction is underway. But with careful calculations and by measuring ahead of time, you can avoid extreme excess. So hand-cut bars are properly recognized as more likely to be untainted and pure than polished, milled bars.

SOAP VERSUS DETERGENT

Soap in its various forms has been used for thousands of years. From the soapy residue of certain herbs, to the potash soaps of yesteryear, to the more refined toilet soaps of today, the limitations of all forms have always been understood and accepted. Only when faced with shortages of fats and oils during World War I did people feel compelled to look for a replacement for soap. This led to the invention of synthetic detergents, but it seems to have led us down the path of no return.

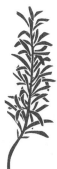

Today we casually toss a cup of soap powder in with our clothing and watch it work miracles. A squirt of blue liquid detergent ahead of time almost ensures a clean-as-new blouse, and a sheet of chemicals tossed into the dryer leaves our clothes soft and floral-scented. Harsh chemicals clean, scent, and coat our clothes. What we may not understand is that many of these synthetic detergents also find their way into our skin-care products.

Soap cleans well in warm, soft, alkaline water, but its effectiveness decreases as water conditions change. When soap reacts with the calcium and magnesium ions found in hard water, it forms an insoluble salt that leaves a residue — a floating curd, or that ring around the bathtub. This compound won't dissolve and is thrown out of the solution, adding to the dirt.

Detergents are more versatile than soap. Though detergents are used most commonly to clean dishes and wash hair, they are also used in combination with soap to make toilet bars, also known as *syndet bars.* Detergent additives, called *lime-soap dispersants,* ensure solubility in all kinds of water. You'll find these additives, listed under a variety of chemical names, on the labels of the most familiar bars of soap on the store shelves.

Although a detergent is loosely defined as any cleansing substance — which would clearly include soap — it more commonly refers to a synthetically derived cleansing product. Detergents are designed to work in the very worst of conditions, and they often do. Once again, however, we pay an unquantifiable price for products that indiscriminately strip clean. Only very harsh, synthetic chemicals clean all materials in all media, and most of our cleaning needs are not so extreme. Perhaps we need to scale down, from overkill to moderation.

NATURAL SOAPS VERSUS SYNTHETIC SOAPS

Perhaps no word has been more overused and more loosely defined than the word "natural." I define it narrowly, a chemist defines it broadly, and most of us have seen so much of it that we're ready to eliminate it.

It is not accurate to define a natural product as one without chemicals — everything on this earth is a chemical. Sometimes it is defined as "organic," but that word is also in the eyes of the beholder. The same is true of the phrase, "no animal products." Some people will not use beeswax because they view it as an animal by-product. (See *veganism* in Glossary, on page 171.)

I define a *natural* soap as one which relies only upon ingredients found in nature for its skin-care qualities. I define a *synthetic* soap as one which relies upon laboratory-made chemicals to make the soap look and feel and act a certain way. All soap has chemical ingredients, but we can think of natural soaps as those made according to natural law, and synthetic soaps as manmade cleaners — synthetic imitations of the real thing.

It's tempting for soap manufacturers to lean toward synthetics and away from natural materials. Synthetics are more stable in more situations. Therefore, they are less expensive in the long run, and — unlike fats and oils which differ slightly from tree to tree, season to season, and region to region — they are the same yesterday, today, and tomorrow. A gram of this chemical, a mole of that one, and voilà — a perfect copy.

As we become more and more comfortable with synthetics in all areas of our lives, we run the risk of losing natural defenses and continually needing greater synthetic intervention. Skin care is but one facet of this phenomenon. Our skin is remarkably capable of functioning on its own to protect us, but, as we use more and more harsh, foreign substances, we alter the body's chemical makeup and leave our skin without its natural defenses. We risk becoming dependent on stronger and stronger synthetics to take the place of the body's natural systems. We must each, as individuals, decide which route to go — the way of nature, or the way of the lab.

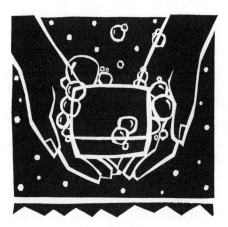

The

Ingredients

PART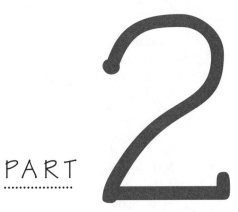

CHAPTER 2
Characteristics of Oils, Fats, and Their Soaps

There are many oils and fats available today for use in soap-making. Only by understanding their benefits, limitations, and availability can you determine which combinations of these are best suited to your particular needs. The essential nature of any soap is directly related to the oils and fats in it.

AVOCADO OIL

Nature: Avocado oil is obtained from the pulp of the avocado pear and is one of the most active and effective ingredients used by the cosmetic industry. Because it has an extraordinarily high percentage of *unsaponifiables* (the portion of the oil which does not react to form soap, but rather retains its original makeup), avocado oil is highly therapeutic. It contains protein, amino acids, and relatively large amounts of vitamins A, D, and E, making this oil very much alive. These components are not only moisturizing, but also healing. They enable avocado oil to regenerate cells, soften body tissue, and heal scaly skin and scalp.

Types/Availability: Avocado oil can be purchased in larger quantities from vegetable oil distributors, or in small bottles at the supermarket or a gourmet food shop. Of course, the smaller quantity is more costly.

Use/Benefits: As with almond oil, avocado oil need not be the predominant oil in a soap formula for the benefits of its qualities to be enjoyed. Don't rely upon this oil for lather or hardness, but instead for its effective unsaponifiables. Splurge and use higher proportions of avocado oil in the base formula in soap for people with extremely sensitive skin.

CASTOR OIL

Nature: The castor oil (sometimes referred to as Palm Christi oil) rendered from the first cold-pressing of the beans is used medicinally. Further pressing yields the grade best suited for soapmaking.

Castor oil's high percentage of *ricinoleic acid,* which gives the oil its high viscosity, sets it apart from all of the other vegetable oils. When calculating the amount of sodium hydroxide required to saponify castor oil, consider the oil's unique make-up. Though it would appear to require less sodium hydroxide, it actually requires more, due to its high ricinoleic acid content. (See page 50 in Chapter 13, The Chemistry of Soapmaking.)

Types/Availability: It is difficult to find local suppliers for soapmaking quantities of castor oil, but many fat/oil manufacturers and distributors carry it in large supply.

Use/Benefits: Like olive oil and jojoba oil, castor oil acts as a humectant by attracting and retaining moisture to the skin. This moisturizing quality makes castor oil well suited for shampoo bars and skin-care products. Castor oil alone is rarely used to make soap because, without other oils, it produces a transparent, soft soap. In combination with other vegetable oils, however, it makes a wonderfully emollient, hard bar of soap.

CAUTION

Though I like the smell of refined castor oil, it has a stronger odor than other vegetable oils. When it comes time to scent a batch of soap containing a high percentage of castor oil, know that the castor oil will overpower your essential oils. The final bars will not necessarily smell of castor oil, but they will carry a diluted, altered form of your chosen scent. You can protect against this problem by simply keeping the amount of castor oil in your formula in balance. Also, raw castor oil has a protein which is a poison. Be sure to buy detoxified castor oil.

COCONUT OIL

Nature: Coconut oil is a gift. It has changed soapmaking more dramatically than any other vegetable oil, and its discovery has led to higher grade soaps. Even companies manufacturing tallow soaps use about 20 percent coconut oil for its lathering and moisturizing properties. Natural soap manufacturers usually combine it with olive, palm, soy, or castor oils for an all-vegetable soap. I cannot say enough about this oil. It offers all soapmaking blends the missing link. Without its wonderful lathering quality, any formula is lacking.

Types/Availability: Today's soapmaker can purchase coconut oil in a few different phases, each phase with a slightly different melting point: 76°F (24°C), 92°F (33°C), 101°F (38°C), and 110°F (43°C), all available in pails, cubes, or drums. The 76°F (24°C) oil begins to solidify somewhere between 72°F (22°C) and 78°F (26°C); the others solidify around their respective temperatures. The coconut oil found at supermarkets is normally the 76°F (24°C) coconut oil. Soapmakers usually have a preference for a particular phase oil based on their particular methods and formulas.

Use/Benefits: Coconut oil is obtained from *copra,* which is dried coconut meat. More than any other fat or oil, it is an anomaly. A percentage of coconut oil in cosmetics is moisturizing. Too much of it can be drying. Its saturated nature resists rancidity and makes a very hard soap, yet its low molecular weight allows for high solubility and a quick, fluffy lather, even in cold seawater.

COTTONSEED OIL

Nature: Cottonseed oil is a by-product of the cotton industry, obtained by steaming the hulled cottonseeds. Though not as costly as some of the more obscure oils, cottonseed oil normally is too expensive for soapmakers to use in quantity.

Types/Availability: Since I know of no manufacturer or distributor that limits pesticide use on cotton grown for oil production, I cannot suggest suppliers. With the many oils available to soapmakers, I urge you to choose one of the others.

CAUTION

One of my personal concerns with respect to cottonseed oil is today's free use of pesticides by the farming industry. Organic farmers are out there, but very few are growing organic cotton. Most of the cotton grown is sprayed with highly toxic synthetic chemicals, and I have concerns about using its by-products in food and cosmetics.

Use/Benefits: Cottonseed oil can be compared to peanut oil with respect to the soap it produces. It is unsaturated, and, though a little slow to saponify with the cold-process, it does offer a quick, abundant, and lasting lather. Cottonseed oil also has emollient qualities, but it is more vulnerable to rancidity than some of the other fats and oils. This is due to a fairly high free fatty acid content, a factor that varies according to the weather endured by the cotton plant after ripening to maturity.

Plants exposed to excess rain and humidity render an oil high in free fatty acids and therefore more vulnerable to spoilage. Watch for this potential problem, which can be corrected by reducing the amount of cottonseed oil in your formula.

LARD

Nature: Lard is obtained by rendering and refining the fat of hogs. Most of us don't understand clearly the distinction between the grades of lard, though the characteristics of the soaps each produces differ enough to make it worth our attention. It's more difficult to place orders for fats and oils if we don't really understand how each one works in our soap formulas.

Types/Availability: Higher grades of lard are edible; lesser grades are inedible. Both are used in soapmaking, though the inedible lard is used more often. The finest lard comes from the fat around the kidneys and has a mild odor. The grades of both edible and inedible lards are no longer clearly defined, and classifications vary from company to company. What once were referred to as choice lard, prime steam lard, and leaf lard, are now known by a variety of names.

Inedible lard is often termed *Choice White Grease,* and, though many soapmakers use it, this grease is associated more with lower grades of soap than the higher grade skin-care soaps. They are made from the less desirable packing house products, and may contain either inedible lard or inedible tallow. They are much higher in free fatty acids than edible lard, so chemical preservatives are often added to delay rancidity.

Most of the fat and oil distributors that carry tallow also carry lard. Some meat processing companies sell lard as a by-product of the manufacturing process.

Use/Benefits: Whichever lard you choose to use, be sure to use it only in combination with some beneficial vegetable oils. Lard will produce a lasting lather, and it does add conditioning and good cleansing qualities, but lard soaps are soft and not easily soluble in cold water. Its skin-care benefits are negligible, and the lower grades produce soaps which, over time, develop a lard odor. So add coconut oil, palm oil, and olive oil to the formula. Better yet, consider the animal rights concern, and stick with the multitude of vegetable oils available.

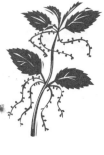

OLIVE OIL

Nature: The first cold pressing of the olive yields the highest grade extra virgin and virgin olive oils. These oils are released from the first gentle pressing of the olive fruit, without heat or refinement (see *refinement* in glossary on page 169). Refined grade A olive oil is obtained by exerting more pressure on the fruit that has already been squeezed lightly to produce the virgin oils. This subsequent pressing, though also cold pressed, contains a higher percentage of free fatty acids and requires some refining. The final pressings of the olives yield what are called grade B refined olive oil and refined pomace olive oil. Grade B refined olive oil is obtained by solvent (usually hexane) extraction using the fruit residue from earlier pressings. Pomace oil is made using the same olive fruit residue used for grade B oil, but it also makes use of the pits (or pomace) of the olives. Each successive pressing is an inferior food grade to the preceding one, but the final pressings are actually best suited for soapmaking.

CAUTION

Watch for adulterated olive oils, where the manufacturer or a distributor has incorporated some cheaper oils to increase profits. An adulterated, name brand olive oil caused me a year of processing problems.

In soapmaking, olive oil often has the reputation of being one of the more difficult oils to saponify, but, with some basic understanding of the different grades of olive oil (see *Types/Availability),* it is as workable as the other fats and oils. It is one of the vegetable oils I consider indispensable and worth the research.

Types/Availability: For years I've been told that, with respect to soapmaking, one variety of olive oil is no different from another: their fatty acid structures, their SAP values, their free fatty acid contents, and their iodine values are basically the same, (see Glossary pages 168–170 for an explanation of these scientific terms). I was told to expect a grade A olive oil, a pomace olive oil, and an extra virgin olive oil to experience the same sort of reaction in the soap pan.

This is just not the case. Within each oil is an unsaponifiable portion. These are the components that don't react with the alkali to form soap. They are thought of as impurities, many of which are removed during the refining process. These unsaponifiables are often overlooked because they're a relatively small percentage of the whole, yet I regard them as a rich source of information about a particular oil, especially each grade of olive oil, because the percentages of unsaponifiables vary greatly from one grade to the next. These unsaponifiables can make one grade of olive oil react very differently from another in the soap pan.

The percentage of unsaponifiables is very high in pomace olive oil, and dramatically lower in a grade A olive oil or an extra virgin olive oil. The unsaponifiables in a pomace olive oil create a thick, waxy, synergistic soup, making the oil more viscous, quick to react, and fast to pull the neutral fats into the soap-making reaction. They act as a catalyst, getting the reaction going and building up some momentum.

Extra-virgin olive oil is the most desirable grade for the gourmet chef, but grades A and B are best suited to the soap-maker who uses a high proportion of olive oil (nearly half of the total oils) in a vegetable-based soap. Pomace oil, with the highest percentage of unsaponifiables, pulls the other vegetable oils into the quickest saponification, but often the pomace oil produces a darker soap, and sometimes overreacts to other soap-making ingredients, particularly fragrance oils, and even some pure essential oils. Fragrance oils, which often contain *dipropylene glycol,* or even certain pure essential oils like cassia and clove, can cause any soap formula to begin setting up too quickly in the pan, but the reaction seems exaggerated in formulas using a pomace olive oil.

For a vegetable soap formula incorporating a high percentage of olive oil, my preference is a grade A or a grade B refined olive oil. If you only have easy access to the higher grades, expect a longer saponification time, or, with a pomace olive oil, be prepared to act quickly once the fragrance is added.

Use/Benefits: Olive oil is a very good moisturizer, not because it has its own healing properties, but because it attracts external moisture, holds the moisture close to the skin, and forms a breathable film to prevent loss of internal moisture. Unlike so many other substances used for this purpose, olive oil does not block the natural functions of the skin while performing its own. The skin is able to continue sweating, releasing sebum, and shedding dead skin. Olive oil, jojoba oil, shea butter, kukui nut oil, and some other natural materials do not inhibit these necessary functions.

I don't choose my soap's ingredients only for the physical properties they lend to the soap. I want each oil to also function as a skin-care product. For this reason, I use a higher proportion of olive oil and accept its more temperamental nature.

Within the industrial setting, where soaps are often milled, olive oil soaps tend to be very hard. Synthetic additives often contribute to this consistency. For the cold-process soapmaker, olive oil (without synthetic additives) does not make a rock hard soap. You must add coconut and palm oils to ensure a hard bar. The color of the final soap varies with the grade and color of the olive oil used, from white to yellow, from light green to dark green. To make a pure white soap, use a grade A or B refined olive oil that looks bright yellow or gold in the bottle.

Though olive oil soaps produce a slow and stingy lather, they are mild and clean well. Pure olive oil soaps, and those made with a high percentage of olive oil and no harsh additives, are generally safe enough for sensitive skin and babies. Castile soap was produced for centuries as 100 percent olive oil soap, though now many companies produce castile bars with part olive oil, part tallow. The boundaries are blurred, and, without ingredient disclosure laws, anything goes, so ask for details on the content of any soap.

PALM OIL

Nature: Palm oil and palm kernel oil come from one variety of palm tree (the oil palm), while coconut oil comes from another variety (the coconut palm). Palm oil is made from the pulp of the fruit.

Types/Availability: Palm oil is harder to buy in small quantity, though suppliers are out there. Not long ago, before high cholesterol was linked directly to saturated fats, palm oil was used by nearly all bakeries. Since we've learned to substitute the healthier unsaturated oils, demand for palm oil is but a fraction of what it once was. Industries other than the food industry use palm oil, but oil and fat distributors do not have the demand to break down tank truck loads (50,000 pounds) into anything smaller than 400-pound drums. However, these companies occasionally are willing to pour a few 35-pound pails while they're pouring a larger order. You must call around and ask. With many calls, you are bound to find someone who is willing to help.

Use/Benefits: A soap made exclusively with palm oil will be brittle and, because of its high percentage of free fatty acids, the glycerin yield is low. In many respects, palm oil contributes many of the same qualities as tallow. They both produce a small and slow lather, and their skin-care contribution is negligible.

Palm oil is wonderful, however, within a mixture of other oils. When it is used in combination with olive and coconut oils, it produces a very nice soap. Though coconut oil produces a fluffy, quick lather and makes a hard bar of soap, we must limit its percentage within a formula to avoid a drying effect on skin. This is where palm oil is useful. It, too, makes a hard bar of soap, and, since it is less soluble in water, its firmness holds up throughout use. It also cleans well, saponifies easily, and is mild. Palm oil is the animal rights advocates' substitute for tallow.

My favorite soaps all include some significant portion of palm oil, because it produces hard bars and speeds up the soap-making process. Palm oil pulls the other soapmaking oils into a quicker saponification. Because the palm oil mixture is more reactive, you must add the essential oils and the nutrients swiftly or the soap will begin to set prematurely.

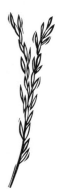

PALM KERNEL OIL AND AMERICAN PALM KERNEL OILS

Nature: There are many palm kernel oils. The oil obtained from the kernels of the African or oil palm tree is the most familiar; this tree bears the fruit used to make palm oil. The oils obtained from the kernels of Central and South American palm trees yield the American palm kernel oils, including babassu oil.

Palm kernel oil and American palm kernel oils contain large proportions of *lauric acid.* This fatty acid is unusual because it combines two mismatched characteristics: saturation and low molecular weight. These traits enable palm kernel oil, babassu oil, and coconut oil to produce hard soaps which also lather well in all kinds of water. Normally, a saturated fat produces a hard soap with weak lathering ability, but these oils also have low molecular weights which produce soluble soaps with easy,

A SOAPMAKER'S STORY
Patricia Arvidson/Island Soap

Pat Arvidson's interest in soapmaking was first stirred in 1977 while she was living in Australia. She saw Ann Bramson's *Soap: Making It, Enjoying It* in a bookstore and thought that making soap sounded like fun. She bought the book, but didn't actually make soap until a couple of years later while living in New Hampshire, and then it was only for her own use.

When her daughter, Jasmine, was born, Pat was living in Deer Isle, Maine. Rather than go back to her nursing job full-time, she decided to try making soap to sell. "I really taught myself how to make soap using a couple of books as a guide," recounts Pat. "I had decided that an all-vegetable soap was the way to go, since I didn't want to contribute to the use of animal products. Through trial and error, and many bad batches, I finally had soap I felt I could sell. I was so excited about my soap in those days, and so believed in what I was doing, that I almost went door to door with my excitement."

Pat's company, Island Soap, offers some wonderful varieties: "Island Seaweed" for a fresh delightful scrub, made with kelp powder, and oils of cedarwood, eucalyptus, lavender, and thyme; "Island Herbal," made with comfrey root powder and a lovely blend of herbal essential oils; "Island Red Rose," made with red clay, patchouli oil, and rose fragrance oil; "Island Bayberry," which is "spicy like the bayberries found here on the island"; "Island Lilac," a pure white bar with the scent of spring lilacs; and bars like Citrus Cornmeal, Spicy Oatmeal, and Coconut Cocoa Butter.

Pat offers a few words of safety advice to all soapmakers. "When Jasmine was just a toddler, she tottled into the soap room (the dining room at that time), saw a wooden spoon with what she probably thought was pudding, and put it into her mouth," recounts Pat. "We rinsed her mouth many times, and she was left only with red spots which healed quickly, but it was pretty scary. Believe me, that was the last time I ever left wooden spoons with raw soap on them lying around."

Reflecting on her soapmaking experience, Pat says, "Through the years, I have really loved making soap — even with all of the bad batches, the late nights, and the challenges of running a business and a family under the same roof. I wouldn't have missed it for anything. I've really loved it."

quick lather. Thus, oils with a high percentage of lauric acid link together the very best of soapmaking characteristics.

Types/Availability: Palm kernel oils are not as common as olive or peanut oil, and you will probably not find them at supermarkets and food clubs. The most familiar palm kernel oil is carried by most fat and oil distributors, and though babassu oil is less common, there are plenty of distributors that sell it.

Use/Benefits: Soaps made from either group of palm kernel oils are white, very hard, and lather beautifully. Though some varieties differ with respect to their melting points, this factor is not important to the soapmaker, who only uses a minority percentage of the oil: 10 to 15 percent is plenty when combined with other vegetable oils. This small percentage also keeps the final bars from developing an odor characteristic of the palm kernel oil. Palm kernel oil, like coconut oil, can have a drying effect when used in excess, yet is moisturizing when used in moderation.

PEANUT OIL

Nature: Peanut oil is made by pressing shelled peanut kernels. Though considered one of the most important oils in the world, its use within soapmaking should be limited to only a minority percentage of the total oils.

Peanut oil is regarded as a non-drying, conditioning oil, offering the softening qualities of olive and castor oils. It is rich in vitamin E and is absorbed well by the skin. Some soapmakers are experimenting with using it in larger quantities, because it is less expensive in bulk than olive oil, but, for all of its benefits as a straight oil, peanut oil soaps are less than remarkable.

Types/Availability: Peanut oil is easy to find: call Oriental restaurants for their suppliers — many are happy to help out; local food clubs carry peanut oil; for very large quantities, contact oil and fat manufacturers and distributors.

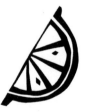

Use/Benefits: Cold-process soaps made from peanut oil are too soft and produce a stable, but weak and slimy lather. However, the addition of palm and coconut oils compensates for its shortcomings. Coconut oil's fluffy, shorter-lived lather, in combination with peanut oil's longer-lasting, fluffless lather, creates a balance. Both coconut and palm oils ensure harder soaps. Also, like olive oil, peanut oil is highly unsaturated. Soaps

containing large proportions of unsaturated oils are more vulnerable to rancidity. Limit the amount of peanut oil to 10 to 20
percent of your total fats and oils.

Once again, maintaining a balance can correct the potential
pitfalls of this oil. By all means, experiment with it.

SOYBEAN OIL (VEGETABLE SHORTENING)

Nature: Soybean oil is the primary ingredient in vegetable
shortening. Soybean oil is extracted from the seeds both by
pressing and solvent extraction. It contains high percentages of
linoleic and *oleic acids,* yielding a fairly soft soap, even in the
hydrogenated state.

Types/Availability: Locate a fat and oil distributor or manufacturer to purchase vegetable shortening in large quantity. Dis-
cuss your soapmaking needs to determine which shortening
will work best. Vegetable shortenings vary from company to
company, with some better for cakes and icings, and others for
soapmaking. Stress your need for hard bars of soap and for a
superior grade of shortening. Local food clubs may offer vegetable shortening in fairly large quantities at a reasonable,
though not wholesale, cost.

Use/Benefits: Though vegetable shortening is often chosen as
a non-animal alternative to tallow or lard, it should be used as
a minority oil in combination with oils which offer better skin-
care properties. Since it is easy to find and relatively inexpensive, vegetable shortening can be used to contribute bulk,
mildness, and a stable lather. Use it in combination with
coconut oil for a fluffy lather, and with olive oil for skin conditioning.

TALLOW

Nature: Tallow has been used in soapmaking more than any
other fat or oil. It is extracted by melting the solid, white, flaky
fat, or *suet,* surrounding the kidneys and loins of cattle, sheep,
and horses. Though soaps have been made for thousands of
years from scraps of fat and reused drippings, most of the tallow that is used in soapmaking today is of a higher grade and
lighter color.

Types/Availability: Only the lighter color grades — which
come either from edible tallows or from the higher grades of

inedible tallow — are recommended for producing a high-grade soap. These contain fewer *free-fatty acids.*

Most of the fatty acids found in a fat or an oil are attached to a *glycerol molecule,* forming a *triglyceride.* Those fatty acids not bonded to glycerol, but instead existing independently, are known as free-fatty acids. They are less stable than the complete triglyceride, and they contribute to rancidity. The higher grades of fats and oils have a smaller percentage of free fatty acids than the lower grades, offering the soapmaker a more reliable material.

The higher grades also have a cleaner odor, though I detect a "meaty" odor while rendering even the finest grades of tallow. I find that even the final soaps made from home-rendered tallow have a meaty odor, which makes them somewhat difficult to perfume.

To render your own tallow, you'll need to find a meat-packing plant or a good butcher to package the suet for you. For large quantity soapmaking, rendering your own tallow is impractical. It requires heating the solid suet with some water and a little salt, eventually yielding cleaner, purer tallow. The process is time-consuming and messy, leaving you with greasy pans and surfaces, even after washing and scouring. It's a bit like plaster dust — it winds up in spots you could swear you were nowhere near. Ann Bramson's book, *Soap: Making It, Enjoying It,* in which she details the rendering process, is a good resource. Try rendering once, but, for long-term soapmaking with tallow, locate a fat manufacturer or distributor that sells pre-rendered tallow in pails.

Use/Benefits: Quite a bit of controversy surrounds the use of tallow in soapmaking. It is thought to clog pores, cause blackheads, and increase the incidence of eczema for individuals with sensitive skin. Tallow's high molecular weight and saturated structure make an insoluble bar of soap with a weak and slimy, though longer-lasting, lather. Tallow supporters point to the wonderfully hard bars it produces, and its ability to saponify (harden into soap) quickly. It is also relatively inexpensive and plentiful. Supporters cite the 5,000 years of tallow use as evidence that it's safe.

Those who oppose the use of tallow do not deny its value to past centuries; they just question its continued use in light of today's alternatives. Some animal rights advocates distinguish between need and convenience: pioneers would not have been able to keep disease under control without using animal by-products to make soap. Their herbal alternatives were far less effective. Today, we have a smorgasbord of vegetable oils to replace tallow in soaps. Many people consider it immoral to kill an animal for a bar of soap, when so many vegetable oils make worthy substitutes. Others argue that animals are sacrificed for their meat and not their by-products, which would only go to waste without soapmaking and other by-product industries. However, the profitability of selling by-products theoretically subsidizes the sale of meat, permitting lower meat prices and encouraging greater meat consumption.

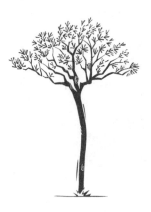

CHAPTER 3
Lye and Water

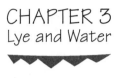

$\mathcal{S}$oaps have been around for thousands of years. Lye, in its present form, was not around throughout most of soap's history. The caustic alkalies (bases) used for soapmaking were potash leached from wood ashes, and various carbonates produced from the ashes of seaweeds and land plants. The soaps were harsh and soft, and often rather unpleasant. Not until the 1700s, when Nicholas Le Blanc discovered a way to make caustic soda (sodium hydroxide) economically, did soapmaking attain new quality levels.

EARLY ROMAN SOAPS

During the first century A.D., the Romans used urine to make a soaplike substance. It contained ammonium carbonate which reacted with the oils and fat in wool for a partial saponification. People called *fullones* walked the city streets collecting urine to sell to the soapmakers.

Lye means one thing to one person, and something else to another. Technically, *lye* has a narrower meaning than *alkali* or *base,* and a broader meaning than *caustic soda* or *caustic potash.* We, as soapmakers, can speak to one another using these words interchangeably, with full understanding of the intent. But to understand the soapmaking process, we must isolate the individual components and learn how each one contributes to the final product.

Lye has two meanings. It is the solid form of a caustic alkali. It is also the water solution in which a caustic alkali has been dissolved. I most often call sodium hydroxide "sodium hydroxide," and the sodium hydroxide/water solution, "lye."

A soap is the neutral product created when the acids of fats and oils react with organic or inorganic bases. Cold-process soapmakers use a variety of fats and oils as the acid, and sodium hydroxide, a caustic alkali, as the base. But many other bases can be used to make soap. The base of choice would depend upon the particular soap. A liquid soap, for example, calls for potassium hydroxide (caustic potash). There are many caustic alkalis, but it is sodium hydroxide which is most help-ful to the cold-process soapmaker.

Sodium hydroxide (NaOH), also named caustic soda, comes in three forms: solid, flake, and liquid solution. Solid caustic soda is impractical for the cottage-industry soapmaker. NaOH predissolved in water is called solution, but, unless the chemi-cal company is local, the cost of shipping the water solution is prohibitive. Flake (or bead) lye is easy to store, easy to find, and easy to use.

Though less expensive in 50-pound bags, I choose to buy sodium hydroxide in 13.5-ounce containers at the supermarket. The Memphis humidity is mighty impressive and finds its way even into well air-conditioned rooms. In the presence of mois-ture in the air, the sodium hydroxide flakes absorb the water and clump into solid chunks. I don't want to go digging for my measurement of NaOH from a solid mass, nor do I want an infe-rior solution. I also have health and safety concerns about stor-ing 50-pound bags of a potentially active chemical in my home. So this is one material I prefer to buy in small quantity. Look for Red Devil plastic canisters at the supermarket, normally shelved next to the Drano. Be careful not to use these inter-changeably. Also, squeeze the can of lye to be sure that the product has not been exposed to moisture or air. A crunchy can should be left behind. For bulk purchases, contact chemical companies. Ask for well-sealed plastic buckets with a poly-ethylene liner.

SAFETY PROCEDURES

Sodium hydroxide is highly reactive in its dry form or within solution. One bead of lye can burn right through layers of skin in the presence of just a hint of sweat. A splash of solution can burn, blind, or at least eat through a butcher block table.

This compound is worthy of our greatest respect and even greater caution. Sodium hydroxide is corrosive to all tissues. Accidentally swallowed, it causes serious internal injury, and it can be fatal. Even the weaker solutions can do extensive damage.

Ingesting lye can be fatal if we do not act immediately. Past literature instructed people to neutralize any ingested sodium hydroxide with acids, like lemon or lime juice, or vinegar, and then to drink a demulcent, like egg whites or olive oil, which often induces vomiting. Poison control centers now urge people **not** to use this procedure and **not** to induce vomiting.

You should check with your local poison control center for the most up-to-date procedures. Be prepared to act should someone ingest sodium hydroxide. As of this writing, the recommended action is to give water only — four ounces for children and eight ounces for adults — and to head to the hospital emergency room. In case of eye exposure, irrigate the eyes with large quantities of running water and seek medical attention. Flood skin burns with large quantities of running water until the soapy, slippery feel disappears, then treat as you would treat any other burn.

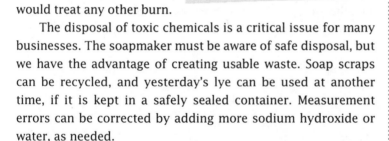

CAUTION

Never dispose of sodium hydroxide, lye, or raw alkaline soap without first researching local landfill regulations. These materials are toxic and hazardous.

The disposal of toxic chemicals is a critical issue for many businesses. The soapmaker must be aware of safe disposal, but we have the advantage of creating usable waste. Soap scraps can be recycled, and yesterday's lye can be used at another time, if it is kept in a safely sealed container. Measurement errors can be corrected by adding more sodium hydroxide or water, as needed.

As your lye cools down for a few hours or overnight, be mindful of exactly where you set down the bowl. Remember to consider children, cats, dogs, and the level of activity in the room. Carefully think through location, as well as all other steps. It's better to cover all bases, even those remote contingencies.

See Chapter 9 for more thorough step-by-step instructions on preparing and using the lye.

MIXING LYE

More than any other one component of your formula, sodium hydroxide must be handled precisely for a trouble-free batch of soap. An ounce or two less or more of water or of a particular oil will not dramatically affect the final soap. But you will notice that difference with respect to the sodium hydroxide. Measure the sodium hydroxide carefully, using a good scale.

Necessary Equipment

Choose a glass or ceramic container for the water. Look for a pitcher with a lip to avoid splashes. Caustic alkalis attack zinc, tin, aluminum, and brass, and the sturdiest of plastics weaken from the heat of the reaction. Some books give the go-ahead to cast iron and steel, but I don't advise using either. At higher temperatures, lye eventually eats away at cast iron, sometimes polluting your solution. Stainless steel seems to hold up better, but, with its high cost, I'd rather earmark those pans for cooking. Finding glass or inexpensive, heavy pottery is fairly simple. A rounded bowl is easier to use than a taller jar.

The mixing of sodium hydroxide and water generates considerable heat; to stir the lye solution, I use heavy-duty rubber or silicone spatulas with heavy-duty plastic handles. Many soapmakers use wood, but day-to-day contact with lye eats into the wood, and before long the utensils begin to splinter off into your solution.

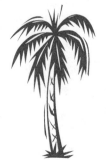

THE ROLE OF WATER

Water is used as a solvent within the soapmaking process. To make soap, three molecules of alkali must react with one molecule of a neutral oil. Dry, caustic soda sprinkled over a mixture of just fats and oils would not come into contact with very many neutral oil molecules, and, in its undiluted form, the sodium hydroxide flakes would be too concentrated for neutralization to take place. Water, the universal solvent, dissolves the sodium hydroxide, carrying it to all corners of the pan. It increases the surface area of the sodium hydroxide, thereby ensuring thorough interaction with the neutral oils.

Water is the only chemically inert component in the soapmaking reaction. Its job is to convert the caustic soda into a usable state, and then to sit tight. The oxygen and hydrogen atoms do not participate in the chemical equation — they remain bonded, as water, even within the final bars. They do not decompose and interact with the other compounds.

Measuring and Testing

The key is to calculate the amount of water necessary to dissolve a specific amount of sodium hydroxide. Too little water won't bring the soda into solution, causing the final soaps to be brittle and dry. Too much water will add unnecessary moisture to the soaps, making them less lasting and too soft. The right amount of water will dissolve the sodium hydroxide, transport it throughout the neutral oils, and add plasticity to the final soaps. Keep in mind that a formula is somewhat flexible with respect to the amount of water required to dissolve an amount of sodium hydroxide; acceptable amounts need not be exact, but rather fall within a range.

Though a soap formula will be somewhat forgiving, hard contaminated water will eventually surface as one defect or another. Hard water contains dissolved mineral salts which are quick to latch on to the sodium hydroxide ions, leaving fewer of the ions to react with the neutral oils. This dilution of the lye saps the solution of some of its strength. Not enough alkali will remain to saponify the full amount of fats and oils.

Test your tap water for softness and purchase distilled water if the results are less than encouraging. The quality of each individual component within your formula is directly related to the quality of your final soap. I occasionally use rainwater, though rainwater may contain many surprises; all sorts of impurities fall into the vessel along with the rain. A bug or two are sure to be floating on top, next to a pine needle, a leaf, and some other unknowns. Always strain fresh rainwater through a strainer lined with layers of cheesecloth.

AN APPRECIATION OF THE SOAPMAKING PROCESS

I sometimes think about those people of past centuries who couldn't run out to the supermarket to buy lye cleanly packaged and ready to use. Just as I'm feeling blessed with convenient and superior products, I'm moved to think hard about those folks. Their lives must have been physically demanding ones, but I wonder whether their days offered greater spiritual rewards.

STARTING THE SOAPMAKING PROCESS

Once the sodium hydroxide has been weighed, carefully add it to the cold water and stir briskly. The fumes will overwhelm you within just ten to twenty seconds. I hold my breath until the beads are fairly well incorporated, and then I leave the room for fresh air. I return two minutes later to completely blend the mixture, being sure to incorporate any sediment which has settled on the bottom of the container.

Let the mixture sit for a couple of hours to cool down. For maximum solubility, be sure to incorporate all of the dry sodium hydroxide in the water while the solution is still very hot. As the solution cools, any excess flakes will harden in a clump on the bottom and make mixing more difficult.

Once cool, cover the lye solution until you are ready to use it. Long-term exposure to air weakens the solution through the formation of sodium carbonate, which forms when the sodium hydroxide combines with carbon dioxide in the air. While pouring the lye into the oils and fats, stir briskly until all of the lye is thoroughly incorporated. Since keeping the molecules in constant contact with one another is what makes soap, try to keep stirring briskly throughout the soapmaking process.

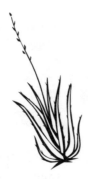

CHAPTER 4
Scents

$\mathcal{S}$centing soap is truly an artform. It can be treated casually as one final, quick step of the soapmaking process, or it can be your very personal *pièce de résistance.* A good bar of soap is one that offers skin-care qualities, but can be experienced sensorially. Notice how the oils glisten once the bar is introduced to water. Let your skin feel the texture of finely ground oatmeal or the silky smoothness of emollient oils. And draw in the blend of scents slowly and deeply. Create your soaps with this in mind.

ESSENTIAL OILS

Many of us feel that we've discovered aromatherapy within the last decade, but the multiple uses for essential oils have been discovered and rediscovered for over 5,000 years. Nearly all essential oils are derived from plants, though a few come from animals: civet from cats caged in farms, musk from the musk deer, and ambergris from whale secretions. A plant's essential oil is somewhat like blood to humans. It flows through the plant's system fighting off disease and predators while attracting beneficial plants and insects.

As soapmakers, when we think of oils, they're usually the fatty oils like olive, jojoba, or coconut. But an essential oil is very different. It is often more like water than oil, as it quickly evaporates once exposed to the air. A plant's essential oil is a unique blend of that plant's characteristics. We enrich our soaps by including these oils and their offerings.

Essential oils are derived from the leaves, berries, flowers, petals, twigs, bark, or stems of plants and usually inherit the scent or flavor of the particular plants. Oils are extracted through distillation or expression, and both methods are tedious and require a sophisticated setup.

Some pure essential oils are very expensive. Massive quantities of plant material often are needed to yield just one ounce of essential oil. Some oils are much more expensive to produce than others because they require so much more plant material

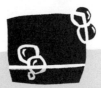

A SOAPMAKER'S STORY

Barbara K. Bobo/Woodspirits Ltd., Inc.

Barbara Bobo of Woodspirits is a medicinal herbalist with experience in aromatherapy. Not surprisingly, then, her soaps are distinguished by their unique combinations of pure essential oils. Woodspirits' soaps are made with a coconut oil/olive oil base; some also include castor and almond oils or lanolin. With names like Seaweed Scrub, Carrara, Phome, and Pacific Mist, these soaps have spicy lathers and gorgeous natural colors. Within the bars are spices like cinnamon and paprika, herbs, and natural pigments, like ultramarine, ochre, chlorophyll, shale, and clay.

The Woodspirits' brochure describes each bar in detail, telling its "story," which makes for fun reading. Azteca, her "ban the bottle" shampoo bar is made with French white clay and spirulina (a simple algae). Portuguese Breakfast Bar, a marbled bar of terra cotta and cream, is made with pure essential oils of bitter almond, cinnamon, petitgrain, and sweet orange. Barley Bath is an "old-fashioned remedy for farm rough hands and wind-chapped cheeks, and homely as a mud fence," made with pure barley flour and fenugreek seeds.

Barbara's soapmaking venture began twenty-two years ago. Today, Woodspirits involves Barbara and her immediate family plus five other families (who are privately contracted for their services), including her brother's family in Nebraska and a father-daughter team in London. Her two sons help with each and every soapmaking, which usually occurs twice a week. They make 480-pound batches and pour the soap into 32-pound molds.

Barbara's business was transformed by a production tip from a gentleman named Reid Worthington, who suggested she use a stainless steel honey vat to increase production from 60 bars at one time to 1,600 bars. "I wasn't sure it would work . . . The morning we made our first batch in that quantity, I was more nervous than I had ever been in my entire life!" relates Barbara. "But it worked beautifully." Reid has since passed away, but, says Barbara, "Thanks to Reid and his unselfish attitude, I have succeeded. I will always remember his kindness, and I will always pass along his idea."

Barbara offers several tips for new soapmakers: 1) Always weigh your lye — don't believe the label; 2) Add the lye to the water, not the other way around, and stir briskly; and 3) Always wear goggles. She also passes on an unusual method they have developed over the years for cutting soap: A hand-operated machine that first used guitar strings and, more recently, aircraft safety wire. Finally, Barbara stresses that honesty, diligence, perfectionism, and — most of all — a sense of humor all go into her soap. "I think it shows," she adds.

for the distillation process, the particular plants are more expensive to grow, and the distillation process is more complicated. For most of us, the pure essential oils of rose, neroli, and jasmine are out of our price range.

Synthetic Oils versus Essential Oils

Synthetic oils often are used to replace the prohibitively expensive essential oils, and, unfortunately, the less expensive ones as well. Synthetic chemicals now recreate just about everything found in nature, but these imitations do not offer the unique properties of the essential oils. For example, essential oils used to soften skin, reduce inflammation, heal a wound, or settle a stomach cannot be created synthetically. An oil absorbed through the skin for its healing quality is valuable only in the essential form. A synthetic reproduction should never be used for aromatherapy.

Some soapmakers swear by synthetic oils and others won't use them. I find that I like one for every fifty that I don't. One company's gardenia oil is lovely, while another's is not recognizable. One honeysuckle oil is true, another is generic. Too many companies create a few "bases" and simply alter them a bit from scent to scent. These oils smell generic and only slightly different than the others — avoid them. Only by sampling and testing various essèntial and synthetic oils will a soapmaker develop a sixth "scent."

Synthetic oils are used most often because they are far less expensive than the essential oils and are less vulnerable to spoilage, since they only contain a small percentage (if any) of

CAUTION

Be aware that even some of the pure essential oils are extracted using chemical solvents which may or may not be completely removed from the final oil. Whenever possible, purchase essential oils which are either cold-pressed or distilled. These are free of residue.

actual plant material. I do find that they are stable on the shelf, but not so stable within the soaps. I finally found a wonderful approximation of tea rose, but then discovered that once in the bars, it spoils after just a few months.

Heat and alkalinity affect both essential and synthetic oils, but the synthetic oils are altered more dramatically by the chemical reaction within the cold-process soap pan. Some completely lose their fragrance and others yield soaps which smell nothing like the oil you poured. The synthetic oils are more prone to begin streaking and then suddenly seize (solidify in clumps) the soap mixture. These oils are often made with dipropylene glycol, or even pure alcohol, which often overwhelms a freshly saponified batch of soap. Also watch for certain pure essential oils, like clove and cassia, that cause the liquified soap to overreact.

Cheap oils can ruin otherwise perfect batches of soap. Large-scale soap production often involves a milling process, where soap is shredded and dried before it is scented, pressed, and extruded into cakes. At the point when this mixture is scented, the soap is far less active and alkaline, and it is more receptive to inferior oils. A freshly made batch of cold-process soap is less tolerant.

OBTAINING ESSENTIAL OILS

More and more companies are offering essential oils and fragrance oils. Because of the complexities of natural oil extraction, there are many more distributors than manufacturers. Synthetic oils are more easily manufactured, so there are more of these companies around. Fragrance companies that also sell pure essential oils are in the fragrance business; they only sell the essential oils used in their formulations. They are not in the business to repackage pure essential oils, and their focus is synthetic formulation, not purity.

Some companies sell nature-identical oils, or natural compound oils, which are not as pure as the essential oils. These are profit busters for these companies; rather than creating a pure essential rose geranium oil using only the rose geranium plant, they tap a few more plentiful plants and combine their similar scents to create a rose geranium-like fragrance.

The closer the distributor is to the manufacturer, the better the pricing. The bad news is that these companies require huge minimum purchases, anywhere from 5 to 8 pounds of essential oil to a full drum or two of each. Further down the line are distributors who will sell you a pound or two of essential oil at pretty good pricing. If you can purchase in larger quantity, do so and avoid the fourth, fifth, and sixth generation distributors who buy way down the line. You pay for the product plus as many mark-ups as there are intermediaries.

Network with other soapmakers and craft businesses to discover the market of suppliers. To qualify for wholesale purchase, you must have a tax identification number. If you are a non-business soapmaker who cannot buy wholesale, be alert to the same discrepancies in pricing within the retail market. These oils can spoil or ice your carefully created formula, so put forth the effort to secure only the most pure and stable scents.

**CONSIDER MAKING
UNSCENTED SOAPS**

Unscented soaps are simply beautiful and the formulas are less temperamental. The most reactive period of the soapmaking process is during and just after the addition of the essential oils. The solution is made less reliable and can overreact. Pouring the soap as is, without adding any scent, minimizes the risks.

STORAGE AND HANDLING OF ESSENTIAL OILS

Essential oils are very different from fatty oils and must be cared for differently. They are very sensitive to light and heat, and evaporate when exposed to air. Store your oils in dark amber glass bottles in a cool area, and keep the caps twisted tightly. Essential oils should not be exposed to temperatures below freezing or above 95˚F (35˚C).

Shelf life varies from oil to oil. Synthetic oils have stabilizers and preservatives so they can last for years. Some essential oils, like sandalwood, patchouli, rosewood, jasmine, and rose, improve with age; others, especially the citrus oils (bergamot, tangerine, lime, lemon, and orange), are vulnerable after just six months. Some people store citrus oils in the refrigerator to extend shelf life. (They must be brought to room temperature before being added to the soap mixture.) Buy fine-quality oils to get the longest life. I have a lemon essential oil on the shelf that's two years old and doing fine, so there are no certainties.

Depending upon how an oil was obtained from the plant and whether or not its integrity was preserved in the process, it may or may not be stable. Most companies advise customers to use up oils within a year, maybe two. I have four-year-old oils which are fine, and I have never had to throw away an oil, but no chart can accurately assign expiration dates. Through use and familiarity, soapmakers get to know their oils. Ask suppliers for their recommendations, but factor in your own experience as well.

Though we should limit chemical intrusion into our soaps, some synthetic oils afford more people a greater selection of scents. In moderation, these synthetic oils can offer value, but be sure to carefully weigh your priorities before choosing a test-tube version of the real thing. Occasionally, I use a synthetic perfume oil, for there are some wonderful blends out there. They do not benefit the skin, however, so use them in moderation and add nutrients to your soaps that do offer skin-care qualities.

Keep in mind that no essential oil has been successfully reconstructed in the lab. Even when laboratory tests reveal a near perfect replica, a synthetic version of a pure essential oil can be identified. A natural oil carries certain intangibles along with its chemical formula.

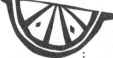

How Much Oil?

The percentages of essential oil used in a soap depend on the formula. When I first learned to make soap, the 12-pound recipe I found called for only a few dropfuls of essential oil. Since I had to work way too hard to detect that scent in the final bars, I added a couple extra teaspoons each time I made a new batch. By the time I was satisfied, a few dropfuls had turned into three ounces of pure essential oil.

Other than people with allergies or those who simply prefer unscented soaps, no one will be overwhelmed by the maximum limit of a pure essential oil carefully blended into the soap. As a fragrance fiend, I want the scent to be an integral part of my soaps. However, each formula does have a saturation limit; a soap mixture can incorporate only so much unsaponified product before separating out the remainder. Using the cold process, essential oils can account for up to two percent of the total weight of a soap's ingredients, though I typically use about one percent. Remember to factor in any superfatting oils, honey, or other natural additives to avoid overloading the mixture. These ingredients are added just before pouring and do not get saponified.

Any excess is visible after the twenty-four-hour setup period once the blankets are removed. Excess essential oil separates out and forms small puddles of oil that you'll find resting on top of a slick mass of hard soap when you open the trays. Such a batch can be salvaged by blotting the solid block of soap and eventually slicing into bars as usual, but the soaps will not be quite right.

The final stages of saponification take place as the soap cures, but an overload of oil throws a monkey wrench into the finish, interfering with the chemical reaction, and altering the final product. The pH can be slightly off, the bars may never harden properly, and the consistency may be somewhat greasy. However, this complication is uncommon and will rarely be an issue if you follow my guidelines.

BLENDING OILS

The following suggestions for blending oils are intended only as a guide; I hope you will use these combinations as a starting point for developing your own scents. Strict adherence to formulas is limiting. No painter would only combine certain colors, and no soapmaker should be constrained by someone else's imagination.

Essential oils are blended to complement one another. They are often more interesting in combination than on their own. However, some work beautifully together and others clash.

The scent of an oil is measured according to intensity: how often and for how long it affects us; whether it "feels" high or low; and its fullness and strength. As you become more familiar with the characteristics of oils, you sense which ones blend nicely and in what proportions. Personal taste will affect your blending choices, but consider the relationship between the oils with respect to these characteristics.

SCENT CHARACTERISTICS OF ESSENTIAL OILS

Fleeting/High/Soft Scents are only briefly detected, but have a sharpness that we "feel" radiate high into our noses. They are the bells which ring out occasionally to emphasize and punctuate.

Steady/Low/Strong Scents are like the kettle drum — the low, steady undercurrent. These oils are slowest to evaporate. They are breathed in deeply and feel full-bodied. They come at us with all they have got, no subtlety and no inhibitions. A little goes a long way!

Fleeting/High/Soft Scents	Steady/Low/Strong Scents
Lemon	Clove
Grapefruit	Juniper Berry
Rose	Myrrh
Lime	Lavender
Tonka Bean	Vetiver
Petitgrain	Patchouli
Neroli	Cedarwood
Chamomile	Ylang-Ylang
Tangerine	Vanilla
Sandalwood	Pine
Bergamot	Clary Sage
Rosewood	Jasmine
Orange	Basil
Geranium	Thyme
	Frankincense
	Nutmeg
	Anise
	Cassia
	Lemongrass
	Rosemary
	Mint

I like to compare the intensity of essential oils to musical instruments and their wide range of expression. Depending upon their pitch, tone, and amplitude, some instruments are arranged to play alternately or in harmony. The same holds true for essential oils. Some oils blend in harmony; others create cacophony.

A kettle drum's noise can be overwhelming if it is not limited. The harp is drowned out by a continuous blast of the saxophone, but if they take turns and balance their volumes, the blend can be rich and harmonious. Bergamot is hard to detect if not enough is used. In the presence of even a little too much patchouli, bergamot will be unnoticeable. When carefully balanced, bergamot and patchouli can be partners.

Patchouli's scent is steady and full. This oil is wonderful as a heady, sensual undercurrent, but too high a proportion of patchouli oil within a blend will overpower the other oils. Be sure to factor in characteristics of all of the essential oils being considered for a blend, using less or more of particular oils depending upon how often, how long, and how fully they will be detected.

The fascinating art of aromatherapy isolates a wide range of characteristics of various oils and assigns relationships between oils and many beneficial properties. For the beginning soapmaker who wants to begin experimenting with essential oils for scent, but is not yet eager to study the science of aromatherapy, my crude, simplified version of scent classifications (at left) will get you started. Also keep in mind that scent classifications within soapmaking are not identical to perfuming combinations, because the sodium hydroxide and the heat affect the blend. If you come to appreciate the essential oils and their beneficial properties, refer to an aromatherapy book for more depth and precision on this topic (see appendix, p.157).

Try to choose oils that balance one another. Choose a high scent to balance a low one, less of a longer-lasting scent to balance more of a fleeting one, and more of a weaker scent to balance a smaller quantity of the strong, full scents. But do not feel compelled to choose your scents in an orderly, rigid fashion. Use these groupings only as a guide, a check-and-balance, to avoid overpowering a blend, and dare to break the rules occasionally for a surprise.

FAMILIES OF SCENTS

Essential oils are also distinguishable by family or type. The following families of oils may help guide you in creating particular blends. Personal preference may lead you toward certain kinds of scents: floral, citrus, evergreen, herbal, fruity, woody, and green. Different scents for different moods — try them all at some point.

Woody	Evergreen	Green
Sandalwood	Swiss Pine	Basil
Cedar	Mountain Pine	Cucumber
Patchouli	Ocean Pine	Violet
Rosewood	Stone Pine	Mimosa
Juniper Berry		

Floral	Herbal	Fruity	Citrus
Carnation	Rosemary	Apple	Lemon
Gardenia	Marjoram	Peach	Orange
Honeysuckle	Dill	Strawberry	Tangerine
Lavender	Tarragon	Apricot	Bergamot
Mimosa	Coriander	Black Currant	Grapefruit
Ylang-Ylang	Juniper Berry	Cherry	Lime
Hyacinth	Fennel		Verbena
Chamomile	Caraway Seed		Petitgrain
Lilac	Clary Sage		
Jasmine			
Rose			
Muguet			
Geranium			
Apple Blossom			
Lily			
Iris			
Jonquil			

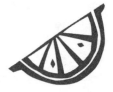

THIRTY-ONE SPECIALTY SCENTS

To scent soap made with any one of the formulas detailed in chapter 9, or one of your own formulas, try the following "specialty scent" combinations of essential oils. To blend a few different essential oils together for a small twelve-pound batch, I suggest you measure by volume instead of weight. You will have more control over excess and waste. Adjust accordingly for larger or smaller batches.

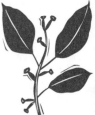

SCENT	OILS	AMOUNT (IN TEASPOONS)*
Citrus	Lemon	9
	Bergamot	5
	Lemongrass	2
	Clove	2
Holiday Spice	Nutmeg	6
	Mace	2
	Cloves	2
	Cassia	4
	Lemon	4
Tuolumne Meadows	Cassia	4
	Lavender	5
	Clove	3
	Caraway	4
	Red Thyme	2
Urania's Gift	Lavender	3
	Lemon	4½
	Rosemary	3
	Sage	3
	Peppermint	3
	Cassia	1½
Oxford, Maine	Sandalwood	10
	Patchouli	5
	Sassafras	3
Carefree Highways	Vanilla	8
	Rose	5
	Sandalwood	5
Steve's Suggestion	Lemon	12
	Almond	6

1 teaspoon = approximately 5 ml

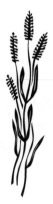

Checkerberry	Cassia	6
	Lavender	12
Pesto	Juniper Berry	7
	Bergamot (or Lemon)	6
	Basil	3
	Patchouli	2
Soft-Spoken	Lemon	9
	Lavender	9
Memphis Blues Bar	Sassafras	4
	Nutmeg	2
	Bergamot	5
	Patchouli	2
	Sandalwood	5
Exeter Street	Vanilla	6
	Lavender	8
	Palmarosa	4
Sassy Soap	Sassafras	5
	Rosemary	3
	Bitter Almond	2
	Lavender	4
	Lemon	4
Sweet Earth	Lavender	9
	Patchouli	3
	Vanilla	6
Summer Spice	Rose	9
	Clove	5
	Peppermint	4
Purple Prose	Lavender	12
	Rose	6
Wipe Away Suspicion	Juniper Berry	7
	Lavender	6
	Rosemary	5
Bar Beatriz	Lemon	9
	Lavender	5
	Rosemary	4
Clean Slate	Sandalwood	6
	Rose	6
	Ylang-Ylang	4
	Patchouli	2
Wash-Your-Hands-of-It	Lavender	5
	Frankincense	7
	Cassia	2
	Rose	4

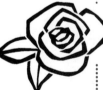

Soap of the Earth	Sandalwood	7
	Orange	3
	Rose	3
	Cassia	2
	Geranium	3
16 Moore Street	Rose	13
	Patchouli	5
Clean-Cut	Geranium	4
	Orange	7
	Lemon	7
Bar None	Sandalwood	6
	Patchouli	3
	Rose	3
	Lavender	2
	Lemon	4
Wipe-Out	Cassia	8
	Sassafras	5
	Bergamot	5
Zabar's Zoap	Cassia	9
	Almond	9
Midnight at Ken's	Caraway	10
	Lavender	5
	Rosemary	3
Plan B	Sandalwood	10½
	Patchouli	4
	Lime	1½
	Clove	2
Bed 'n Breakfast	Cassia	4
	Rose	5
	Clove	4
	Bergamot	5
Allegheny Adventure	Lemon	8
	Clove	4
	Sassafras	6
Southern Summers	Ylang-Ylang	4
	Vanilla	4
	Tonka Bean	4
	Lime	6
The 11th Hour	Juniper Berry	6
	Red Thyme	5
	Lavender	4
	Rosemary	3

ALLERGIES

People react adversely to all kinds of materials, including the most natural. We, as soapmakers, are alert to synthetic allergens, but we also must think of pure essential oils as potential irritants.

To the best of my knowledge, no one has ever had a problem with my soaps. Cold-process soaps made with minimal alkali are rich in glycerin, emollient oils, and unsaponifiables. These soaps are far more pure than their synthetic counterparts and people with sensitive skin can count on their simplicity.

Within a cold-process soap, essential oils account for only a small percentage of the total materials, and most people do not react to such dilution. However, there are people who cannot be exposed to a drop of fragrance within a skin-care product or in the air. These are the same people who have come out in droves requesting fragrance-free magazines; they are not just a handful of individuals. They are allergic to fragrance and cannot tolerate even the more subtle essential oils. For these individuals, we must offer unscented soaps, using no fragrance and mild fatty oils.

Someone who is sensitive to essential oils may react to any one of the many varieties of essential oils, but experience has shown a few scents to be more of a problem than others. Be alert to the oils that are potential allergens, but know that I have used many of them liberally in my soaps over the years without a single complaint, even from people with sensitive skin.

OILS THAT MAY BE POSSIBLE IRRITANTS

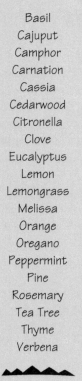

Basil
Cajuput
Camphor
Carnation
Cassia
Cedarwood
Citronella
Clove
Eucalyptus
Lemon
Lemongrass
Melissa
Orange
Oregano
Peppermint
Pine
Rosemary
Tea Tree
Thyme
Verbena

A SOAPMAKER'S STORY
Camille Le Doux/Camille Le Doux's Handmade Soaps & Toiletries, Ltd.

In the 1890s, Camille Le Doux's great-grandfather, Marcel Majeau, owned a pharmacy on Bourbon Street in New Orleans where he made and sold soaps and toiletries to the French opera singers. Marcel Majeau was well known among the gentry for his wonderful handmade "Savon au Bouquet" (scented soap). He used pure olive oil and lye in his soap. As a port city, New Orleans had easy access to exotic essential oils, like rose and jasmine, which Mr. Majeau incorporated into his soap. "One of his most interesting recipes which I still make today is Sportsman's Soap," says Camille. "It contains citronella, a natural mosquito repellent herb, and Litsea Cubea, a naturally deodorizing, lemony herb. Another trick of his that I use is to put ground cinnamon into my soap. It smells heavenly and it gives soap a wonderful marbleized appearance."

Camille's great-grandfather taught his daughter, Louise Majeau, how to make his soap, and Louise, Camille's grandmother, passed along her knowledge to Camille. Though Camille still makes many of his soaps, she substitutes a combination of coconut, olive, soybean, and almond oils for the pure olive oil, which she can't obtain as inexpensively as her great-grandfather could. Living in Cajun country where soybeans grow, Camille finds a plentiful supply of soybean oil, to which she adds coconut oil to make the soap lather better.

Camille's soaps include "Voodoo Spice," which incorporates frankincense, myrrh, jasmine, curry, and marjoram, an herbal soap for dry skin, and an almond soap for oily skin. She incorporates into the soap pure essential oils, like rose, jasmine, and lavender, as well as powdered frankincense and myrrh, and — from her garden — aloe vera and rosemary (which she throws into the food processor before stirring in).

Camille makes her soap in 25-pound batches in her kitchen, pours it into airtight plastic containers, and lets it sit for two weeks. After removing the block of hard soap from the containers, she lets it sit for another week, and then cuts the block into four-ounce bars with a metal spatula.

CHAPTER 5
Colorants

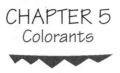

When it comes to personal care products, sometimes we get caught up more in the presentation than the usability and convenience of the product. Some guest bathrooms are spotless, with beautifully embroidered linen towels lined up on the counter, and multi-colored soapballs, polished and dry, sitting on a china plate at a safe distance from the sink. Such special touches are welcoming, but they can also scare people away from using anything for fear of ruining the effect. We want our skin-care products to be inviting and usable, not just for show.

Bright, multi-colored soaps are often more artful than useful. Avocado green, deep rose, and vibrant lavender soap colors are created in the chemist's lab, and with these beautiful shades come the health risks of using synthetic chemicals. Synthetic dyes are used to color everything from food to cosmetics to medications, and yet too much of what is approved for safe use has not actually been proven to be so. They carry some very real carcinogenic risks. When it comes to coloring soap, my advice is to leave the test-tube neons to the painter's palate, and allow the earth's offerings to color your soaps naturally and safely.

Once you've gone to such extremes to ensure a pure product using only the finest materials, why compromise just to make your soaps look like everyone else's. My advice is to use only the ingredients which add desired properties to your final bars, and to leave out those that are just for appearance's sake.

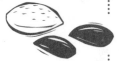

SYNTHETIC VERSUS NATURAL OPTIONS

Until the 1850s, only natural coloring was available for dyeing. For thousands of years, people relied upon vegetable, plant, and animal dyes, as well as mineral pigments. Then, in 1856, an Englishman accidentally produced a pale purple dye called mauve. Natural dyes have now been replaced almost entirely by these synthetic dyes. Coal tar, a by-product of the coal industry, is used to make synthetic dyes. We know these from our labels as D&C (drug and cosmetics) and F, D, and C colors (food, drug, and cosmetics).

The FDA limits the percentages of lead and arsenic allowable within these dyes, but many suspected carcinogens are not taken off the market. We, as consumers, are left to assess purity. This is a heavy responsibility, and one which I try to evaluate product by product. At the very least, I know that I can control what goes into my soaps.

Scale down your expectations for soap coloring, and you will be pleasantly surprised. Muted earth tones are not gray and dirty looking: The colors of Yosemite are quiet and natural, yet vibrant. Aim for this effect within your natural soaps.

Lye and coloring battle one another for control of the soap's final appearance, and the lye wins. Milled soaps retain a richer color because the soap is flaked, dried, and stabilized before the dye is introduced. In cold-process soapmaking, the coloring is added right before pouring into the mold, while the soap is still active and caustic. Within this solution, the colors are altered and paled and rarely look anything like their original state. Go with the flow, and be ready to be surprised, knowing that your soaps will be unique and safe.

I have never used candle or other synthetic dyes, but I have had fun experimenting with natural alternatives. Vegetable dyes like beet juice, cherry juice, or blueberry juice, which I used successfully in creating lip balms, were a flop in the soap pan. What a dull, gray mess they made once introduced to the all-powerful lye. Ground spices are wonderful. They add scent, texture, and deep earth tones. Herbal infusions and decoctions rarely keep their original color, but usually create something interesting. Mineral pigments are effective, but this is one natural product I choose not to use. Other soapmakers swear by them, but I have safety concerns (see page 56). Caramel, cocoa, oatmeal, cornmeal, chlorophyll, carrot oil, annatto seed . . . we have many natural choices!

GROUND SPICES AND HERBS

Ground spices are particularly fun to use for coloring, as they also add scent and texture. Powdered cinnamon is a favorite, but try cloves, nutmeg, and allspice as well. The soaps they

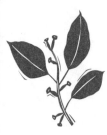

produce are speckled and range anywhere from a caramel color to a dark chocolate. Curry powder and turmeric yield shades of yellow and peach, and I'm told that saffron does as well, though the cost keeps me from playing with it in soap. Cayenne pepper and paprika create beautiful, salmon-colored soaps. All of these are made even more interesting by marbling the color throughout the soap mixture, leaving swirls of color against a contrasting background.

Rather than adding the spice powder directly to the soap, which can result in clumping, first beat it into a small amount of the soap mixture or into a tablespoon of avocado or olive oil, and then add that mixture to the larger batch. Experiment with the desired degree of color, from 1 tablespoon (15 ml) of spice up to ¼ cup (59 ml). If you increase the amount up to ½ cup (118 ml) for a 12-pound (5.45 kg) batch of soap, you run the risk of spicy lathers and a heavy-duty cleanup job.

HERBS FOR DYEING SOAP

Lady's Bedstraw (roots and flowers)
Alkanet (leaves and root)
Goldenrod (flowerheads)
Saffron (blossom)
Indigo (leaves)
Woad (blossoms)
Annatto Seed
Nettle (leaves)
Elderberry (leaves, berrries)
Yarrow (flowers)

HERBAL INFUSIONS AND DECOCTIONS

You can make a concentrated herbal infusion using powdered or chopped leaves or flowers combined with mineral water. The amounts of each are variable, though I'd recommend starting by pouring 2½ cups (591 ml) of boiling water over 8 to 12 ounces (227 to 340 g) of plant material. Let the mixture steep for six to eight hours in a tightly covered glass container, then strain thoroughly. This preparation can be made up to a day in advance and stored in the refrigerator.

Making a decoction from roots and bark requires a more intense process that involves soaking and then simmering the plant's tough parts. Begin by cutting or crushing the roots, bark, or seed into small pieces and soaking them in cold water for ten minutes. Pour the mixture into an enamel or glass saucepan and slowly bring it to a boil. Reduce heat and simmer for ten to fifteen minutes, or until the mixture is reduced to about a quarter of its original volume. Cover tightly to prevent evaporation and allow to steep for five to ten minutes more, then strain thoroughly. Refrigerate until ready to use, no longer than twenty-four hours.

Use either the infusion or the decoction in place of an equal amount of water for dissolving the lye, but expect a less stable color than you'd achieve with a synthetic dye. Experiment, and enjoy the off-tones you achieve. None of the herbs listed in the box can be counted on to produce a particular color. Too many factors come into play: the combination of oils and fats, nutrients, and essential oils; the amount of sodium hydroxide used; and even which day of the week it is!

PLANT OILS, PLANT EXTRACTS, AND VEGETABLE COMPOUNDS

Olive oil, castor oil, palm oil, and wheatgerm oil, which enrich your soaps, will also provide a gentle tint. The essential oils of carrot, patchouli, vanilla absolute, and cassia bark, used primarily to scent soaps, add some coloring as well.

A variety of plant extracts can also be used to color and enrich soap, but since they aren't all oil-based, each extract must be researched individually. Ask for oil-soluble extracts, and do not use the water-soluble extracts which incorporate propylene glycol. You should also research the method of extraction used to avoid unwanted synthetics. Annatto extract, grapeskin extract, and beet root extract offer shades of red (and other surprise colors depending upon the soap formulation), but be sure to order the pure oil-soluble extracts.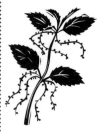

Vegetable compounds produce some natural colors. Liquid chlorophyll tints soaps a natural, pale shade of green. Caramel, a gently burnt sugar, offers warm earth tones. I've heard that hydrated tomato colors soap a shade of red, although I haven't tried it myself.

In coloring, remember that part of the soap's beauty is its unadulterated makeup.

INORGANIC MINERALS

Minerals mined from the earth are called inorganic because they were never alive. Most minerals form within extremely hot liquids deep inside the earth. As the liquids cool, some of the atoms bond together to form crystals. Over time, more and more layers of atoms attach themselves to this unit, forming ever-growing crystals.

Minerals are among the first substances used by humans, but their use in soapmaking concerns me. Though many cosmetic manufacturers, including the natural companies, use mineral pigments, I am not convinced of their safety.

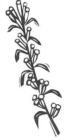

Mica, shale, pumice, ochres, titanium dioxide, iron oxides, and ultramarine seem to be used safely by many reputable soapmakers. Just be on the alert to some of my concerns. Mica and pumice contain free silica, which, in excess, has led to respiratory diseases. Ochres (or ochers) — mixtures of sand, clay, and iron compounds like iron oxides — are thought to be safe unless the iron oxides are ingested. Titanium dioxide, another metal oxide, is also thought to be non-toxic, unless the titanium oxides are inhaled in massive amounts. Ultramarine should not be thought of as the genuine article of long ago derived from the gem lapis lazuli. Today it is made by heating a mixture of kaolin, sodium carbonate, sulphur, silica and resin to very high temperatures. Note that any of these minerals can cause skin irritation: the natural versions are filled with impurities, and the synthetic versions are exposed to some unfavorable catalysts.

Pearlescent Pigments

Many soapmakers are using striking pearlescent pigments to decorate their soaps. Pearlescent pigments are microscopic, transparent layers of mica coated with titanium dioxide or iron oxide, and arranged in parallel layers. As light is absorbed and reflected through these layers, we see flashes of glitter and pearls, called pearlescence. The particular transparent colors we see are determined by the thickness of the titanium dioxide or iron oxide layers coating the mica. Iron oxide reflects the deeper bronze colors and titanium dioxide reflects the brighter earth colors.

Though natural titanium dioxide and iron oxide *may* be relatively safe, once the impurities have been removed, the particular forms of titanium dioxide and iron oxide used to make pearlescent pigments are created synthetically in the lab — the pure oxides are not as easily applied to the mica as the synthetic versions. Also, the strict rulings limit the use of the pure oxides within cosmetics. To achieve the brighter colors, synthetic colorants are added to many of the pearlescent pigment formulations.

Some companies sell a natural version of their synthetic pearlescence, using guanine crystals obtained from herring scales. Read safety data sheets carefully; guanine is often suspended in a highly synthetic base. If it is, this is not a natural alternative.

Many minerals have been found to be toxic only under conditions that soapmakers are unlikely to experience. We will not be inhaling or ingesting large quantities of these materials, and yet I don't want to absorb anything through the skin that would be toxic to other systems. I just don't feel comfortable with the depth of the research done, and to me, the benefits are not great enough to justify the potential hazards. I prefer to let the skincare materials within the soap formula color the final bars ever so slightly with natural tones.

A long history does not make something safe. We have misused natural substances for thousands of years, and then claimed purity because of their longevity. People have always lightened, darkened, and colored their faces and bodies as fashion dictates. From ancient Egypt to modern America, we have paid more attention to the effect than the result. In the name of beauty, people have whitewashed their faces, adorned their bodies and faces with lead paints, and covered blemishes with toxic paints and dyes. Men and women in 18th century England wore make-up daily. The lead paints were toxic and left people looking old in their twenties. Some people died from lead poisoning.

My recommendation is to leave the mineral pigments for pottery and keep them away from our skin, which readily absorbs the good and the bad.

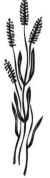

A nutrient is an ingredient included in your formula not only for its ability to make soap, but also for its skin-care properties. Some nutrients are emollient, others are conditioning. Some stimulate the skin, others heal it. A few nutrients protect the other ingredients from spoilage while offering the skin vitamins, and attracting moisture. Many soaps are drying, but organic nutrients can reverse this, creating a soap that cleans gently and moisturizes.

Some nutrients, like oatmeal, aloe vera, or chlorophyll, are added to the soap mixture right before pouring. Coconut, castor, avocado, sweet almond, and olive oils work a double shift. They are nutrients, but they also participate in the saponification reaction.

Any ingredient which saponifies can either be included in larger quantity from the start of the soapmaking process, or added in small quantity just before adding the essential oils. For example, evening primrose oil will saponify and can be used as a major soapmaking oil to replace a portion of one of the other oils, but most people find it too costly to use in large quantity and instead add a few tablespoons (4 tablespoons [59 ml] per 12-pound [5.45 kg] batch) at the end of the soapmaking process. Too much liquid incorporated at the end of the soapmaking process will separate out of the bars later on.

Though a large amount of a nutrient offers the greatest benefit, even a smaller quantity added at the end will enrich your soap. The basic soap recipe should already be filled with beneficial soapmaking oils like olive, coconut, and avocado, so these few tablespoons of added nutrients are an extra dose. When nutrients are added after the soap has saponified, they will remain unsaponified within the final bars, making a superfatted soap.

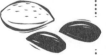

SWEET ALMOND OIL
Use/Benefits: Almond oil, obtained from the dried kernels of the almond tree, is an excellent emollient, known to soften, soothe, and condition skin. It is easily saponified and produces

a very mild soap with a nice lather. Since it is quite expensive, almond oil usually accounts for only a small percentage of the total oils used within a formula.

Quantity/Procedure: A little goes a long way though, and a relatively small amount is needed to make a superior soap. This nutrient can be saponified in large quantity as a soapmaking oil included from the start with the other oils, or 4 tablespoons (59 ml) per 12 pounds (5.45 kg) of soap can be added just before the essential oils.

ALOE VERA

Use/Benefits: The sap or gel found within aloe vera's succulent leaves is an effective healing agent for the treatment of burns, injuries, and acne. This cool, clear gel is soothing and moisturizing, as it stimulates the growth of new cells and tissue with steroids, enzymes, and amino acids.

Quantity/Procedure: To incorporate aloe vera gel within soap, add 4 tablespoons (59 ml) to a 12-pound (5.45 kg) batch just before adding the essential oils. Be sure to use only fresh, pure aloe vera gel, as synthetic preservatives or additives destroy its cellular properties. Even following all precautions, be aware that the heat of the cure period is likely to rob the aloe vera gel of some of its curative powers.

Caution: Note that some people find the fresh aloe vera gel irritating — I am one. It can sting and itch, so test the gel first on a small patch of skin before using it in your own soap.

AVOCADO OIL

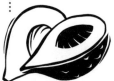

Use/Benefits: Avocado oil is therapeutic. It contains vitamins A, D, and E, protein, carbohydrates, amino acids, chlorophyll, and glycerides of many fatty acids. It also has a high percentage of unsaponifiables — those portions of the oil which do not break down during saponification and are thought to have softening properties. Our skin easily absorbs avocado oil and responds well to its healing quality; it is known to regenerate skin cells and soften tissue.

Quantity/Procedure: Replace a portion (one-quarter to one-third) of your fats and oils with avocado oil, or thoroughly incorporate 4 tablespoons (59 ml) of it per 12 pounds (5.45 kg) of soap just before adding the essential oils.

BALSAM COPAIBA

Nature: Some confusion surrounds this natural oleoresin, tapped from trees in the Amazon rain forest. It is said that Amazon natives have long used this "sap" to heal and soothe. Companies are advertising balsam copaiba (pronounced co-pa-ee-ba, co-pay-ba, or co-pie-ba) and copaiba oil (the oil derived from the copaiba balsam) to heal wounds and soften skin.

I am intrigued by the history of this natural gift, but I am not sure of its skin-care properties. For years it has been used as an organic motor fuel; within paints, varnishes, plastics, and photographic processing; as a diuretic and laxative; and as a fixative in scenting soaps and perfumes.

Use/Benefits: As I research this oleoresin and the oil, their chemical makeups read more like that of an essential oil or a fixative than a fatty oil (in the opinion of a layperson). They seem well-suited for use as scents or fixatives: like tea tree oil, balsam copaiba and the copaiba oil could be used to scent cosmetics with a pleasant, woody fragrance; they could also be used as a fixative within cosmetics, perfumes, soaps, and lotions.

Though balsam copaiba may offer skin-care qualities, robbing the trees of this resin depletes their source of life, and, in time, they die. I opt for one of the many other healing sources, since this one can't be replenished.

CALENDULA OIL

Nature: Calendula, also known as pot marigold, is an herb whose blossoms yield calendula oil, known for its skin-care properties. For therapeutic benefits, be sure to use only the pure oil extracted without solvents.

Use/Benefits: Calendula oil's regenerative and anti-inflammatory properties are known to successfully heal a variety of damage. The oil promotes the healing of wounds, burns, and tissue, and softens and soothes dry, chapped skin.

Quantity/Procedure: Add 4 tablespoons (59 ml) for every 12 pounds (5.45 kg) of soap just before adding the essentials oils. Since calendula oil will saponify, it can be included from the start as a replacement for a portion of the other soapmaking oils, but it is expensive to use in large quantities.

Confused regulations have blurred the classifications of some ingredients; calendula oil may be listed as calendula extract. Be sure to ask for the oil-soluble extract, and not the extract made with propylene glycol.

CARROT ROOT OIL, CARROT SEED OIL, AND WHEATGERM OIL
Use/Benefits: Look for vitamin-rich carrot and wheatgerm oils where you purchase high-grade pure essential oils. Each of these oils offers particular vitamins, and, depending upon your specific needs, they all discourage spoilage and soften skin. Wheatgerm oil (which is very high in vitamin E) inhibits oxidation within the unsaponified portion of your soap. It also contains carotene and vegetable lecithin which nourish skin cells and prevent moisture loss.

Carrot seed oil is high in beta-carotene and vitamin A, and carrot root oil is a highly concentrated blend of vitamins A, E, and provitamin A. Vitamin A heals dry, chapped skin, and both of these oils are good antioxidants. They also stimulate the sweat glands and the sebaceous glands, which work to balance the skin's moisture content. The carrot oils are expensive, particularly the carrot root oil, but a little goes a long way and they are effective.
Quantity/Procedure: Use these oils in quantities no less than .5 percent of the total ingredient weight for satisfactory results. I have used as much as 5 percent for maximum benefit. Add these vitamin oils to your fats and oils just before the lye is added, being sure to thoroughly incorporate them. Adding them toward the end of the soapmaking process is an option, but their antioxidant properties are maximized when the vitamins can have direct contact with the fats and oils — the potential sources of rancidity.

CASTOR OIL
Use/Benefits: Castor oil, like avocado oil, is active within your final soaps. This thick, viscous oil is soothing and lubricating, and is absorbed quickly by the body. In its presence, other, less easily absorbed materials are more likely to be absorbed. This is an advantage if the other ingredients are pure and therapeutic. However, be aware that castor oil is indiscriminating and will just as readily carry a synthetic substance into our systems.
Quantity/Procedure: Either replace a portion (.1 to .2 percent) of your total fats and oils with castor oil or thoroughly

incorporate 4 tablespoons (59 ml) per 12 pounds (5.45 kg) of soap just before adding the essential oils. Too high a percentage of castor oil will produce a soft, transparent soap.

CLAY

Nature: Clays are combinations of finely ground minerals found within the earth. There are many clays, but most are too harsh to be used in a skin-care product. Out of the universe of clays, perhaps a half dozen are occasionally used in soaps. The two most common are kaolin and bentonite. They contain silica, aluminum, iron, calcium, magnesium, zinc, and potassium.

Use/Benefits: Clays are used in skin-care masks to draw out excess sebum, toxins, and dirt. A clay clears the pores of blockages and encourages a more regular flow. This leaves the skin more receptive to natural moisture, yet free of excess. I am somewhat skeptical, however, about the effectiveness of clay in soap. Given the very diluted presence of clay in a soap bar, and given that the lather is rinsed off quickly, I question how much waste it could absorb.

A few soap manufacturers are adding clay to their soaps for its astringent and cleansing qualities. Clays are thought to clean all types of skin, though they seem best suited for people with oily complexions. I find them too drying for combination and dry skin when used regularly.

Types/Availability: Of the many clays available, each one contains its own unique combination of minerals. White clay, or kaolin, contains a high percentage of the mineral kaolinite, and is used within a variety of cosmetics. It is the most pure of the clays; the others are often colored artificially. Green clay, or bentonite, also known as montmorillonite or French green clay, contains a high percentage of mineral montmorillonite. Bentonite has a slippery feel, can absorb large quantities of water, and is the clay typically used in a face mask. It stabilizes the production of sebum and cleans the skin.

Quantity/Procedure: For those who want to experiment, add the clay to your soap just before pouring into molds, using ½ to 1 cup (118 to 237 ml) for a 12-pound (5.45 kg) batch of soap.

Before adding the pure essential oils, blend the clay with 2 cups (473 ml) of soap mixture in a small container. Then blend this clay/soap mixture with the remainder of the batch, stirring briskly. Proceed with the scenting, if desired.

Caution: Minerals derived naturally by ingesting a well-balanced diet offer the skin what it needs to function normally. The minerals we dig from the ground may also draw out waste, but I have the same concerns about these that I do about mineral dyes: the minerals' purity and suitability for skin care are in question.

Clays contain silicates and free silica, which both are suspected of causing health problems. When silica is not bound to other minerals in the form of a compound, it is called "free" silica. It is this unbound silica which is thought to be hazardous. Potters who are exposed over time to these materials have experienced a variety of illnesses, from shortness of breath to an increased incidence of infections, and cases of silicosis, a condition with asthma-like symptoms.

Kaolinosis, a "clogging" of the lungs from inhaling large quantities of kaolin dust, is also caused by the "free" silica within these minerals which enters the lungs and never breaks down. New lung tissue grows over this free silica, and as more free silica is inhaled and more lung tissue forms, the lung eventually chokes from the build-up.

Topical use is very different from inhalation, yet I don't want to absorb any material through the skin that is toxic to my lungs. I don't feel that the long-term effect is well enough understood to take the risk.

EVENING PRIMROSE OIL, BORAGE OIL, AND ROSA MOSQUETA ROSEHIP SEED OIL

Nature: Evening primrose oil, derived from evening primrose flowers, contains a high content of linoleic acid and, more important, gamma-linolenic acid. The small, oval fruit inside the rose bud is called the rose hip, and the oil from one particular species, the Rosa Mosqueta rose, yields an oil rich in essential fatty acids — called Rosa Mosqueta rosehip seed oil.

Borage oil, the essential oil derived from the leaves of the borage plant, has even higher percentages of gamma-linolenic acid. The human body does not produce these essential fatty acids (also known as vitamin F), so we must be sure to include these nutrients in our diets and skin-care products.

Use/Benefits: Essential fatty acids are unique because they offer the skin and the entire body a wide range of benefits. Evening primrose, borage, and Rosa Mosqueta rosehip seed oils are easily absorbed by the skin, encouraging the transport of these essential fatty acids.

Essential fatty acids inhibit bacterial growth and encourage the production of antibodies, enabling our systems to defend against infection and inflammation. They also combine with protein and cholesterol to build membranes which link cells to one another. Water loss, resulting in eczema, hair loss, and dry skin, is thought to be related in part to low levels of essential fatty acids. Vegetable oils with high percentages of essential fatty acids ease inflammation and itching, moisturize the skin and scalp, and treat scaly skin and dandruff (see definition of essential fatty acids, page 167). These three oils are best suited for dry skin and shouldn't be used by people with oily complexions.

Quantity/Procedure: Though they can be saponified as high-percentage soapmaking oils, the high cost is limiting. A little goes a long way though, so add 4 tablespoons (59 ml) of either oil to 12 pounds (5.45 kg) of soap, just before adding the essential oils.

JOJOBA OIL

Use/Benefits: Jojoba oil is actually a liquid wax which solidifies below 50°F (10°C). Its ability to offer the traits of an oil and a wax makes jojoba effective within oils, creams, butters, shampoos, and soaps. Be sure to buy pure jojoba oil and not a synthetic imitation, or you forfeit all meaningful skin-care properties. Jojoba oil resists rancidity and is, therefore, highly stable within soap as an unsaponified, superfatting material.

I use jojoba oil in my creams, shampoo bars, and some of my soaps. Within each product, it serves as a moisturizer and a *humectant.* The skin and scalp benefit from its greaseless lubrication and its ability to hold in natural moisture while attracting external moisture.

Healthy skin receives a regular flow of sebum which lubricates and softens the skin, and traps bacteria that we later wash away with soap. Jojoba oil contains more than four times the waxy esters found within human sebum. When our skin's system is pushed past its limits, jojoba oil helps us maintain normal functions while allowing the skin a chance to repair and rebalance. A thin breathable layer of jojoba oil can regulate the flow of our natural sebum while controlling evaporation and dryness.

Quantity/Procedure: Add jojoba oil as a percentage of the total soapmaking materials during the initial mixing of fats and oils, or incorporate 4 tablespoons (59 ml) of it per 12 pounds (5.45 kg) of soap just before adding the essential oils. For a superior product, do both, but be aware of its high cost. Also, should you choose to use jojoba oil to replace a portion of the fats and oils, make note of its very low SAP value and adjust the sodium hydroxide accordingly (see page 153, "SAP Value Chart to Calculate Sodium Hydroxide").

KUKUI NUT OIL

Nature: The kukui nut tree is the official state tree of Hawaii. Within its fruit are the nuts and kernels from which kukui nut oil is expressed. For hundreds of years, Hawaiians have used this nongreasy oil to treat sunburns and chapped skin. Kukui nut oil is high in linoleic and linolenic acids — essential fatty acids which are critical for healthy skin — and it is easily absorbed by the skin.

Use/Benefits: Research has shown kukui nut oil to benefit acne, eczema, psoriasis, sunburns, and chapped skin.

Quantity/Procedure: Kukui nut oil is expensive, but a little goes a long way. Even 4 tablespoons (59 ml) added to 12 pounds (5.45 kg) of soap just before incorporating the essential oils adds richness to your soaps. A higher percentage of kukui nut oil added to the other base oils is even better — 10 percent of the total oils makes an outstanding soap.

OATMEAL/HONEY, CORNMEAL, FLAX SEED MEAL, JUNIPER BERRY MEAL, ALFALFA MEAL, JOJOBA MEAL, FLAKED SEAWEED

Nature: Our skin needs to be cleaned periodically of impurities. As skin functions normally, sweat glands and sebaceous glands rid our bodies of waste and toxins. They also trap external pollutants on the skin's surface in a barrier of sebum and sweat. It is our job to clean the slate regularly.

Exfoliants are materials with irregular textures used to release debris which collects on the skin's surface. They add some texture to our soap's lather, increasing the soap's cleansing qualities: the grainier lather removes dirt and dead skin cells while stimulating the healthier cells below. Always include some moisturizing nutrients (sweet almond oil, shea butter, jojoba oil) within this formula to avoid irritation and dryness. When using exfoliants, never rub with force. Soap and a little texture will pick up much debris, without a heavy hand.

Use/Benefits: Oatmeal, cornmeal, flax seed meal, juniper berry meal, alfalfa meal, flaked seaweed, and jojoba meal can all be added to soap for texture. Oatmeal, jojoba meal, and alfalfa meal exfoliate gently. Juniper berry, flaked seaweed, and flax seed meals are more coarse, with sharper edges; finely grind them before adding as exfoliants to soap.

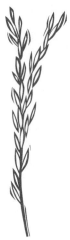

My favorite soap is an oatmeal/honey soap. The oatmeal gently scrubs away debris while the honey hydrates and soothes the skin. Honey is also moisturizing and it inhibits the growth of bacteria. Warm the honey slightly in a bowl of warm water (not hot) to increase solubility. Because its active ingredients are destroyed in the presence of high temperatures, incorporate the honey just before adding the essential oils.

Quantity/Procedure: ½ to 1 cup (118 to 237 ml) of meal is suggested for a 12-pound (5.45 kg) batch of soap, though these amounts are dictated by personal preference. Add exfolients immediately after the soap has saponified. Stir well to avoid clumping, or add the meal first to 2 cups (473 ml) of the soap mixture in a separate container, then incorporate the soap/meal mixture back into the full pan of soap.

To make an oatmeal/honey soap, first blend in the oatmeal, then incorporate no more than 4 tablespoons (59 ml) of warm honey for a 12-pound (5.45 kg) batch of soap, and finally add the essential oils. Blend these swiftly and thoroughly, to avoid an overload of liquid and a quick setup within the soap pan.

Seaweed flakes, particularly of lithothamnium calcareum, can be used as an exfoliant within soap. See following entry about seaweed and its beneficial properties. Blend in 1 to 2 cups (237 to 473 ml) of flaked seaweed per 12 pounds (5.45 kg) of soap just before adding the pure essential oils.

SEAWEED (ALGAE)

Nature: There are thousands of species of seaweed, and many have been used within cosmetics for their nutrients. Since blood serum and seawater are so similar, chemically, many of the vitamins and minerals we need are found in seawater and sea plants: from vitamins A, B, C, D, E, F, and K to iodine, magnesium, copper, zinc, iron, calcium, phosphorus, nitrogen, and manganese. Seaweed has many more vitamins and minerals than land plants. It offers therapeutic properties: seaweed attracts and retains moisture, making it an excellent humectant; it is used for cell regeneration, to soothe and heal the skin; and it acts as an antioxidant.

Use/Benefits: Unfortunately, seaweed does not readily release its nutrients within cold-process soapmaking. Seaweed, as flakes and flour, should be added for texture and design, but do not expect these pieces to contribute meaningful nutritive value within a bar of soap. Seaweed extracts do offer the concentrated nutrients, but only in a water-soluble or a propylene glycol base, and neither is well-suited to cold-process soapmaking.

OTHER EXOTIC BUTTERS

As you experiment with using shea butter in your soap, you may want to also investigate other exotic butters such as Dhupa, Kokum, Mango, Mowrah, Sal, and Illipe.

SHEA BUTTER

Nature: Shea butter, also known as African karite butter, is expressed from the pits of the fruit of the African butter tree which grows in Central Africa. This butter has been used for food and body care. It is remarkably high in unsaponifiables, up to 11 percent, making it a superior superfatting material for soapmaking. Unsaponifiables are those components within the fat or oil which do not decompose and combine with the sodium hydroxide to form soap, thus remaining in their original state within the bars, able to moisturize and nourish the skin.

Use/Benefits: Shea butter is gentle enough for babies and people with sensitive skin. It soothes and softens dry, chapped skin, while nourishing all skin types. I have come to rely heavily upon shea butter for its effectiveness.

Quantity/Procedure: Add shea butter (2 to 5 percent of your total fats and oils) at the start of the soapmaking process to the still-warm coconut oil, then add this combination to the other vegetable oils. To incorporate it at the end of the process, incorporate 4 tablespoons (59 ml) of shea butter — melted and cooled to approximately 75°F (24°C) — just before you add the essential oils.

ECODERMINE

Sederma, a company based in France, and one of the first to introduce shea butter, has patented a product called Ecodermine, which is a combination of glycerin and sugar alcohols. Ecodermine was designed to balance the skin's "microflora," a community of resident (beneficial) and parasitic microorganisms: the resident flora can digest the sugar alcohols and multiply; the parasitic flora cannot digest these sugar alcohols, and are even thought to be slowed in their presence, inhibiting this population.

Environmental factors, use of harsh cosmetics, and over-cleansing can reduce the beneficial flora, enabling the parasitic flora to multiply quickly and stake its ground, leaving the skin defenseless. Ecodermine is designed to feed the skin's beneficial bacteria, leaving less room for outside parasitic microorganisms that dry and expose the skin to the elements.

Sederma suggests using 1 to 5 percent Ecodermine in soaps, but the cold-process soapmaker will have trouble incorporating any amount of Ecodermine at the beginning of the soapmaking process because the lye will probably destroy the integrity of the product, leaving few, if any, beneficial properties within the final bars. A few tablespoons incorporated at the end of the process may be of little benefit to the soaps. Because Ecodermine is a relatively new product, there is little research to evaluate, but I encourage you to follow the continuing reports as to its effectiveness. The initial studies are intriguing.

A SOAPMAKER'S STORY
Jane Hawley/Nature's Acres

With a degree in horticulture and twelve years specializing in growing and selling herbs, Jane Hawley now creates personal care products that incorporate organically grown plants and their medicinal properties. "We hope you can feel the love and respect for our earth and its rejuvenating power as it flows from our gardens to you," Jane writes to her customers. Her company is located on 130 acres in Baraboo Bluffs, Wisconsin, thought to be the site of the oldest quartzite in the world, formed perhaps one and a half billion years ago.

Drawing on the bountiful harvest of the surrounding fields and woodlands, Jane uses herbs, almond and olive oils, beeswax, vitamin E, aloe, comfrey root, and pure essential oils like melissa, patchouli, rose geranium, lavender, and peppermint in her soaps, bath salts, body oils, lip balm, toner, salve, and moisturizers. Her skin-care soaps incorporate the healing herbs she grows: Peppermint-Aloe Soap, a stimulating, astringent bar with healing properties; Rosemary-Oatmeal Soap for deep cleansing; Lavender-Vitamin E Soap to repair overexposed skin and act as a milk deodorant; and Almond-Sage Scrub, a gentle exfoliant with an antiseptic quality. All of these soaps are colored only with the speckled colors of the dried herbs.

Jane passes on to other soapmakers two creative adaptations she's developed: for soap frames, she has designed removable sides which can be pulled apart from the bottom piece to allow easy access for cutting the bars; as a great cutting tool, she uses an L-shaped piece of galvanized metal, first brought to her attention by her five-year-old son when he was rummaging in the basement.

CHAPTER 7
Preservatives

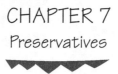

Decay is inevitable. We can slow it, but we cannot stop it. A preservative is defined as something that protects against decomposition, yet nature dictates that everything must decompose. As we fight nature by using preservatives, we may kill off some bacteria and slow further growth, but even the more potent preservatives do not stop decay.

Shelf life, more than well-being, has come to dictate a product's ingredients. A skin-care product is expected to weather all sorts of contingencies. It may sit in inventory for a few months. It may travel and then sit in someone else's inventory. It may sit on the shelf in a store for six months, and the consumer may not open it for three more months. Manufacturers demand years of stability from these products, and add enough synthetic preservative to ensure a long shelf life. But research has shown that the bacteria continue to grow, it's just that the more potent chemical preservatives, colors, and fragrances camouflage the decay. We don't benefit from true purity, yet we suffer the effects of indiscriminating toxins.

As soapmakers, we can control what goes into our soaps. We can choose to use no preservative and allow our soap its fullest potential — and limitation. We can use natural preserva-

---

SYNTHETIC PRESERVATIVES TO AVOID

- Formaldehyde (in the form of MDM Hydantoin)
- Imidazolidinyl urea (known as Germall)
- Phenoxyethanol (phenol and phenolic compounds)
- Captan
- Boric Acid
- Hydroquinone
- Triclocarban
- Irgasan DP 300
- Alkyltrimethyl ammonium bromide
- BHT (butylated hydroxytoluene)
- BHA (butylated hydroxyanisole)
- Calcium Disodium EDTA
- DHA (Dehydroacetic Acid)
- TBHQ

tives which add nutrients to the soap while gently discouraging spoilage. Here too, we must accept eventual decay, but still offer a superior product.

Alternatively, we may choose synthetic preservatives, which may offer the longest protection of all but with a great price. The list of known carcinogenic preservatives is growing. Our skin, which so readily absorbs borage oil, also absorbs toxins. A preservative strong enough to kill some bacteria will also kill our skin's beneficial bacteria. Finally, the active nutrients so carefully chosen for their ability to interact with cells, tissue, and the environment are rendered less effective, if not inert, in the presence of the more potent synthetic preservatives. The choice is ours.

Though I provide a list of synthetic preservatives to definitely avoid, I discourage the use of all synthetic preservatives, and therefore do not offer instructions for their use. All of my research has discouraged me from experimenting much with synthetic preservatives, so I'm not comfortable making recommendations about any of them.

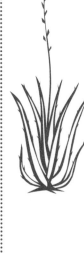

NATURAL PRESERVATIVES

Since the ideal preservative does not exist, I choose natural preservatives knowing their limitations and expecting only what is reasonable. They extend the shelf life of the soap by a few months, without altering the other ingredients and without causing allergic reactions. They also offer skin-care qualities.

People are eager to be educated about natural products and their strengths and limitations. You will be pleasantly surprised to see how receptive others are to relearning what to expect from their skin-care products. Once people understand what makes a natural product more pure and safe, they are willing to accommodate its peculiarities. They learn to purchase smaller quantities and use up the product before buying more. Should a bar spoil (which is not common), they accept occasional throw-aways as the price for purity and safety.

Cold-process soaps are more vulnerable to spoilage than soaps made by other methods because they are normally superfatted (made with excess oils) for mildness. Toward the end of the saponification process, the lye is used up before all of the oil, leaving some oil out of solution in the final bars. This free fat is moisturizing and soothing, but it also causes deterioration. In solution, oils are more stable.

Free oils and nutrients like aloe vera and honey are active ingredients, beneficial because they have living properties in the final bars of soap. As these ingredients complete their life cycles, decay is inevitable, a fact we must understand and appreciate.

Selecting a Preservative

A soapmaker selects a preservative for its antioxidant and antimicrobial properties. When oxygen molecules are able to break their bonds and travel freely throughout an oil or a fat, they combine with other molecules, thus altering the structure of the soap. This is oxidation, the first step toward spoilage, discoloration, and a decrease in nutritive value. As oxidation takes place, soaps will show visible signs of spoilage; small, yellowish circles will appear, just one at first, with more appearing on the soap's surface over a number of weeks. An off-odor follows the first circle of rancidity.

Antioxidants greatly reduce this process by pairing with the "loose" oxygen molecules, rendering them less destructive, and therefore prolonging the useful life of our soap. Antimicrobial preservatives slow down the growth of bacteria in soap, but they cannot prevent it.

There isn't a rigid formula for determining which natural preservatives and how much of each to add to your soap; many factors influence their effectiveness. You need to experiment to determine what works best within your own particular soap-making formula.

The most helpful book I've read on this subject is *Natural Organic Hair and Skin Care,* by Aubrey Hampton, an authority on natural, organic cosmetics, and founder of Aubrey Organics. Over the years, he and other researchers have tested a variety of natural preservatives, including pure essential oils, citrus seed extracts and oils, vitamins, tocopherols, and carrot root oil. His results are exciting and compelling. I now include a combination of a few of these nutrients in my soaps, and the shelf life has been extended by months. My average bar is now good for a year. Longer than a year is more than we should expect from a natural product.

A few observations: Citrus oils are prone to rancidity; ascorbic acid, water-soluble vitamin C, is nearly impossible to find in a non-synthetic form, and it also overreacts to the sodium hydroxide within the lye solution, turning the lye dark and unpleasant; the oil-soluble form of vitamin C, ascorbyl palmitate, which can be incorporated into the fats and oils, is always synthetic; and retinol, naturally derived vitamin A, has practically been replaced with a synthetic version. The natural form of retinol is occasionally available, but the cost is prohibitive.

WHAT CAUSES RANCIDITY IN SOAP?

Rancidity is related to many other factors. Unsaturated oils and fats are usually more prone to rancidity. A mild soap, using the minimal amount of sodium hydroxide for a not quite complete saponification, will have excess fats or oils which do not saponify. These superfatted soaps are gentle and mild, but they also spoil more quickly. Soaps and raw soapmaking materials which are exposed to heat or light will spoil sooner. High percentages of synthetic fragrance can also affect a soap's stability. A humid environment accelerates deterioration.

A Few Recommendations

Grapefruit seed extract and carrot root oil used in combination offer vitamins A and C and skin-care qualities in a non-synthetic form. If your formula is vulnerable, look toward a combination of grapefruit seed extract, tocopherols (vitamin E), and carrot root oil. These are the three natural preservatives I prefer.

Some of these preservatives are added to the oil phase (the mixture of oils and melted fats) of your soap and some to the water phase (the combined and cooled mixture of sodium hydroxide and water). Some are antioxidants, while others discourage bacterial growth. A carefully designed combination can offer your soaps a broader protection from rancidity.

GRAPEFRUIT SEED EXTRACT

Nature: This is a by-product of the citrus industry and is my most reliable antioxidant for soapmaking. Made from vegetable sources, grapefruit seed extract contains vitamin C (ascorbic acid) and glycerin. It has a seven- to nine-year shelf life.

Use/Benefits: Along with its antioxidant properties, grapefruit seed extract is also antibacterial, antimicrobial, deodorizing, astringent, and antiseptic.

Quantity/Procedure: Add between .5 and 5 percent (of the total soapmaking ingredients) grapefruit seed extract to the oil phase before adding the lye solution. Note that the grapefruit seed extract would precipitate out of the lye phase — I learned this first hand.

TOCOPHEROLS

Nature: These are naturally derived forms of vitamin E, existing as either alpha-tocopherol, beta-tocopherol, gamma-tocopherol, or delta-tocopherol. The gamma- and delta-tocopherols are known for their antioxidant properties.

Use/Benefits: Tocopherols can delay rancidity within certain soap formulas, and they secondarily offer healing properties, thereby softening dry skin. Avoid dl-alpha-tocopherol, the synthetic version of vitamin E.

The addition of tocopherols is most effective in preserving tallow and lard, which are low or deficient in natural tocopherols. They also help to protect the more vulnerable essential oils like lemon, orange, and grapefruit. Vegetable oils already have varying percentages of tocopherols, so additional tocopherols may add only a small benefit.

Quantity/Procedure: When using them in all-vegetable soaps, combine the tocopherols with grapefruit seed extract for greater protection. Be sure to use natural tocopherols, not the synthetic reproduction. Add .06 percent (of the total soapmaking ingredients) to the oil phase before adding the lye solution.

CARROT ROOT OIL

Use/Benefits: Like grapefruit seed extract, carrot root oil is an excellent substitute for the pure forms of vitamins C and A, which are becoming more and more difficult to buy in their natural states. Carrot root oil is an antioxidant, high in vitamin A, vitamin E, and provitamin A. This oil is especially good for dry, chapped skin, as it accelerates the formation of new cells.

Quantity/Procedure: Add .5 to 5 percent (of the total soap-making ingredients) carrot root oil to the oil phase before adding the lye solution. Combine with other natural preservatives for greater protection.

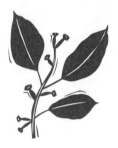

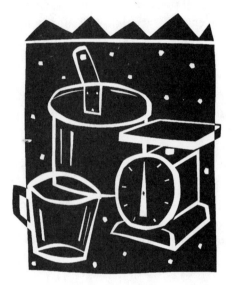

Making

Soap

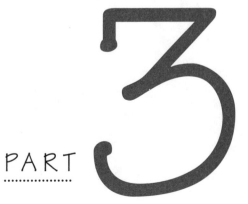

CHAPTER 8
Getting Started: Equipment and Supplies

▼▼▼▼▼

$\mathcal{S}$oap can be made using millions of dollars of equipment or in a bucket. I have settled on the following list of supplies after years of experimentation with all sorts of other options, choosing these for precision, convenience, economy and durability. You will surely have your own ideas, as you venture through soapmaking. Play with them all — that's half the fun.

Ideal soapmaking equipment includes:

◆ 8–12 quart enamel or stainless steel pot with lid (the "soap-making pan")
◆ 3 quart (2.8 liter) saucepan
◆ 2–3 quart (1.9–2.8 liter) heat-resistant glass bowl or pitcher
◆ 2–3 heavy-duty rubber or silicone spatulas
◆ Good quality scale (preferably two scales — one measured in grams and one in ounces)
◆ Two good quality thermometers (0˚–220˚F [18˚–104˚C], quick-read best)
◆ Molds (1 wooden tray 25½"x13½"x4" [64.8 cm x 34.3 cm x 10.2 cm] for a 12-pound [5.45 kg] batch)
◆ Heavy-duty waxed paper for lining the trays
◆ Masking tape to flatten paper against the sides of the tray
◆ Sharp, thin paring knife for cutting and trimming soaps
◆ Safety goggles and gloves

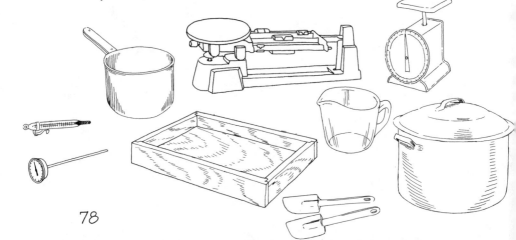

EQUIPMENT MATERIALS TO AVOID

Soap may be fairly harmless and mild, but its components go through some very active, caustic stages before they are tamed. Equipment for the soap-making process must hold up to these components at their nastiest. Lye eats through some materials instantly, and others over time. Cold-process soaps are free of their caustic properties only after weeks of curing, so the equipment used, from beginning to end, must weather varying concentrations of lye. Here are my recommendations of materials to avoid.

◆ Do not use anything made of aluminum, tin, iron, and teflon, which are all corroded by lye.

◆ Avoid cast-iron; seasoned iron pots deteriorate somewhat, discoloring the soap.

◆ I find plastic too weak and flexible in the presence of high temperatures, although heavy-duty plastic is better.

◆ I avoid wood. After using wooden spatulas for a couple of years, I switched to heavy-duty rubber or silicone spatulas, since the wooden spatulas become soft, splintered (leaving tiny splinters in the soap pan), and impossible to thoroughly clean when constantly exposed to the caustic soda. Rubber or silicone spatulas are more expensive, but are good as new two years later.

Heat-resistant glass, earthenware, heavy-duty rubber (white), silicone, enamel, and stainless steel all hold up well to the powers of lye. I use all of these except for stainless steel. It is very expensive, and I save these pots and utensils for cooking only. But if you happen to run into an old industrial stainless steel pot at a flea market, grab it. From thermometers to spatulas, from lye pitchers to the soapmaking pot, try to locate the materials I've recommended since they are the safest and most durable.

SCALES

A year or so into soapmaking, I relaxed about the precision of my measurements, but I've returned to more precision. The cold-process soapmaker must be especially accurate because the process does not allow for adjustment later. Once the lye is poured into the oils, the cold-process soapmaker has no reliable way to correct a little more of this or a little less of that. At best, this method produces soaps which are either slightly superfatted or slightly alkaline; our preference is clearly for the slightly superfatted, which we must ensure through careful measurement.

A NOTE ABOUT MEASURING

Do not measure ingredients by volume (except for essential oils, which can be measured by either volume or weight). Weight is far more reliable. A couple of soapmaking manuals offer formulas calculated by volume, but unless you're feeling confident with this system, it's worth recalculating the formula (carefully) into weight.

Some ingredients are measured most precisely on a gram scale; others are too heavy for the non-industrial version and are weighed accurately enough on a scale measured in ounces. For over a year, I weighed all of my ingredients in ounces, but most of these scales have two-ounce increments, leaving it up to you to approximate the one-ounce and half-ounce measurements. Fats and oils can be measured accurately enough this way, but with respect to sodium hydroxide, essential oils, and natural preservatives, an ounce off is significant. So I keep both scales on hand and consider it a worthwhile inconvenience to switch back and forth.

While my orientation is primarily toward the Imperial system of measurement used in the United States and the Fahrenheit scale for temperature, I realize some readers may prefer metric measurements and the Centigrade scale. For these readers I have included conversion measurements in my recipes.

MOLDS

I am less knowledgeable in this area than many soapmakers are, since I prefer a simple chunk of soap over fancy shapes. A few years back, I played with seashells, cookie molds, and soapballs, and though they were fun for a time, I drifted right back to cubes and rectangular chunks of natural, dense soap. I don't even like the bevelled look, so I save myself the time and the effort of extra cutting.

If you want to experiment with molds, look past the obvious. Once you open your mind to possible receptacles, the strangest objects begin to catch your attention. Textured ashtrays, plastic cookie trays which are divided into decorative compartments, well-scrubbed seashells, children's toys, plastic wine glasses . . . let your imagination go. This is the fun part. Ceramic and glass molds often don't release the soap, lending themselves as soap dishes set beside a sink for dabbing. Plastic and rubber can be gently pulled from the final soap, leaving the shapes intact.

Cold-process vegetable soaps made without palm oil will probably be too soft to satisfactorily mold. They make better soapballs than detailed sculptures. A formula incorporating 25 to 30 percent palm oil will be firm enough to mold, though tallow soaps are the ones best suited to decorative molding.

Wooden Trays for Bars

For rectangular bars, I use wooden trays made from 1-inch plywood with tightly sealed and mitered corners, and handles attached to the sides for convenience. If made well, these hold up for years. My trays measure 25½" x 13½" x 4". Using the formulas in this book, this size tray yields 40 bars, each about 1 inch thick. These measurements don't have to be exact, but if your tray dimensions are different, expect slightly thinner or thicker bars. The important variable is the number of square inches in the bottom of the tray — in my case, 344 square inches. The depth is not as critical, except that less than four inches doesn't accommodate heavy-duty waxed paper as comfortably. You can also make trays from heavy cardboard boxes, but they warp quickly and need frequent replacing to avoid uneven bars.

I always line trays with heavy-duty waxed paper to avoid deteriorating wood and subsequent soap discoloration. My trays are only slightly higher than the height of my bars, a most efficient height for conserving heat during the twenty-four-hour insulation period. I cover one tray with another, upside down tray, and then wrap both well with blankets.

Some very costly industrial frames come with inserts for dividing the mass into bars. I have not found an inexpensive alternative for vegetable soaps. While the addition of palm oil leaves a fairly hard soap within just 24 hours, deep inside the bars the soap remains soft for longer than you'd want to leave them in the molds. I find it's better to slice the bars and let them air dry with the softer parts exposed. This method works best for me, and people do love hand-cut bars. Again, working with a 100 percent vegetable formula is very different from working with a tallow formula, though worth the initial inconvenience.

SAFETY EQUIPMENT AND CONCERNS

Everyone, especially beginners, should wear goggles and gloves as a safety precaution.

Purchase gloves that are somewhat close-fitting, allowing you a degree of feel. Look for latex, neoprene/latex, heavy plastic, or natural rubber gloves. Make sure that the material is not slippery; it's important to have a reliable grasp.

As you decide how to handle the safety issues for you, your family, or any unknowing passers-by, keep in mind the dangers of dry sodium hydroxide, the lye solution, and even the less concentrated soap within the pot. Pots and bowls should not be placed close to the edge of a counter or a table. Consider cats and dogs; educate your family; put up warning signs; make sure that you will be able to monitor the process from start to finish or wait for another time; and factor in all sorts of contingencies before deciding to proceed.

THE WORK AREA

The beauty of soapmaking is that anyone can make soap in almost any setting. The process is flexible and adaptable to a variety of arrangements. Even the few requirements which must be followed can be creatively satisfied. Most of my suggestions stem from the fact that sodium hydroxide in any form is potentially dangerous. The other suggestions relate to the convenience of making soap within easy access of the stove, the sink, and the ingredients themselves. Carrying pots of sloshing oils from room to room and carting around supplies is a messy nuisance.

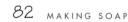

Selection and Setup

People make soap everywhere — from the basement, to the garage, to the kitchen, to the barn. Very few have tailor-made studios to satisfy all soapmaking needs. I use my kitchen because everything is accessible, and I can have the family nearby. (Anyone who chooses to be centrally located must educate the family.)

Soap can be made way out back in a barn without power, exposed to the elements, and far from the soapmaking ingredients (which should be stored inside at room temperature to avoid early rancidity). To be on the safe side, however, and for convenience and a more stable product, try to find a place that meets basic requirements.

Ideally, the following guidelines should be considered in choosing a work area. They are listed in order of importance.

1. A stove should be located within a few feet.
2. A sink should be located within a few feet.
3. Ingredients and supplies (sodium hydroxide, oils, scales, and utensils) should be stored within a few feet.
4. The workspace should be counter height with enough area (approximately 50 square feet) to spread out all the equipment and the ingredients. Avoid wood and metal; my butcher block island in the kitchen has some battle scars.

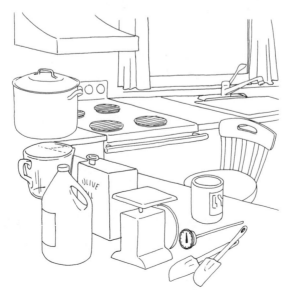

5. Room temperature should be moderate, not under 60°F (16°C) or over 95°F (35°C). Again, this is ideal, but even extreme temperatures can be dealt with creatively.

6. Locate a comfortable chair to accommodate the height and depth of your work area.

Some people bake from the hip and others measure and set out all of the ingredients beforehand. The soapmaking process accelerates quickly, so you're more likely to succeed if the ingredients and supplies are sitting there waiting for you. Plan time to set up your area and equipment well before you actually make soap. First cover the work area with heavy cloth or newspapers. Then line the soapmaking trays and weigh out all ingredients that can be prepared ahead of time, as detailed in the instructions for making soap in Chapter 9.

CHAPTER 9
Recipes

Soap can be made with less precision than the following formulas suggest, but the beginning soapmaker should start out being exact. Experimentation and study will eventually allow for creative license.

Soaps made with a high percentage of beef tallow (half of the total amount of fats and oils in a formula) can be made with a wider range of temperatures than vegetable oil soaps. But, soaps made using only vegetable oils, or even those which are mostly vegetable oils incorporating a small percentage of tallow or lard, should be made at close to 80°F (27°C).

Personal preference may eventually lead you toward 90° to 95°F (32° to 35°C), but even a 15-degree increase creates a whole new set of challenges. All-vegetable oil mixtures can take much longer to saponify at temperatures between 95° and 105°F (35° and 41°C); they may curdle between 100 and 140 degrees (38° and 60°C), even with regular stirring; the lye can precipitate out of solution into solid little pearl-like pieces which wind up as solid lye in the final bars; vegetable soaps are more vulnerable to rancidity when they are produced at higher temperatures; and temperatures below 75°F (24°C) and above 95°F (35°C) produce a mixture which overreacts to scent.

For the first year in business, I made vegetable soaps (from olive oil, coconut oil, and vegetable shortening) very differently than I do today. I used much less sodium hydroxide than the recipes called for, leaving a much higher percentage of unsaponified oil in the final bars. The soaps were more vulnerable to early rancidity, but they could be made slowly over a sixteen to

A NOTE ON TEMPERATURE
The processing temperature affects the length of time it takes for soap to saponify. I recommend a processing temperature of 80°F (27°C). In my experience, as the temperature climbs from 80°F to 100°F (38°C), the processing time increases by ten to thirty minutes. Above 110°F (43°C), the processing time speeds up again, but the soap becomes less desirable.

twenty-four hour period, allowing for a very leisurely process. I brought both the lye solution and the oils to 95° to 100°F (35° to 38°C), combined the two, and then stirred down the oils into the mixture every so often, as they separated like oil and vinegar. At bedtime, I could just cover the pan, go to bed, and stir down the oils in the morning.

This process allowed me some flexibility, but it does not work well with palm oil, tallow, or a pomace olive oil, which speed up the soapmaking process, and ultimately I decided to choose the hard bars produced by palm oil over the leisurely soapmaking process.

You, too, will probably change formulas over the years, as half the fun and the challenge involves some experimentation. Read all you can to understand soapmaking fundamentals, but then take off in your own direction.

The fourteen recipes in this chapter can be used to create dozens of other recipes using the various nutrients described in Chapter 6. Read about the nutrients and their skin-care qualities, then design your own soap formulas which best suit your particular needs.

BASIC STEPS OF THE SOAPMAKING PROCESS

Step 1: Set up the soapmaking equipment, including scales, a soapmaking pan, a saucepan, thermometers, a glass bowl, and ingredients. Measure out the essential oils, preservative, and extra nutrients; set aside in separate containers.

Step 2: Line the soapmaking trays with heavy-duty waxed paper, keeping the paper 1 inch from the top of the trays on all sides. Mitre the corners, one at a time, by pushing your forefinger along the paper and pressing deeply into the corners, using your other hand to keep the rest of the paper flat and in place.

Step 2

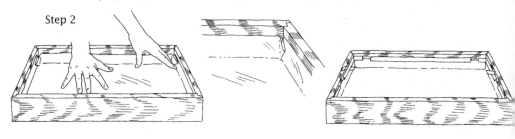

Gather the excess paper in the corners inward to form flat hospital corners. Flatten the folds perfectly flush against the frame and secure with masking tape, from the bottom corner out diagonally to the exposed area of the frame. Tape the edges of the paper to the box at intervals to keep the paper flat against the frames, without waves and wrinkles, and to prevent forming soaps with rounded edges and wavy bottoms. Do this now — you won't have time later as things speed up.

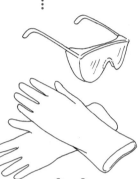

Step 3: Put on safety goggles and gloves.

Step 4: Weigh out the sodium hydroxide and set aside, away from the work area.

Step 5: Set a 2-quart glass container on the scale; weigh out required amount of water.

Step 6: Carefully add the sodium hydroxide to the glass container of water, stirring briskly with a rubber spatula until it is completely dissolved.

Step 3

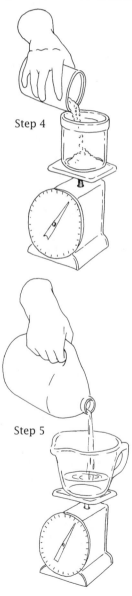

Step 4

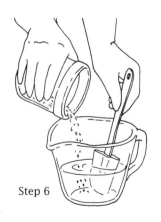

Step 5

Step 6

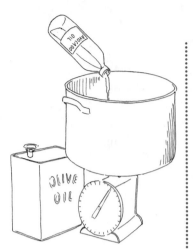

Step 7

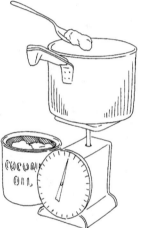

Step 8

Step 7: Place the 8 to 12-quart soapmaking pan on the scale. Add the required weights of the liquid soapmaking oils that are to be included at the start of the soapmaking process. Set aside.

Step 8: Place the 3-quart saucepan on the scale and weigh out the solid fats that are to be melted before being added to the liquid oils. Set aside.

Step 9: Wearing goggles and gloves, slowly drizzle the lye into the oils, stirring the mixture briskly.

Step 10: Continue to stir briskly, circling the pan and cutting through the middle of the pan with your spatula to keep as much of the solution as possible in constant motion.

Once a small amount of soap drizzled across the surface leaves a trace pattern before sinking back into the mass, the soap is ready.

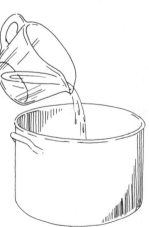

Step 9

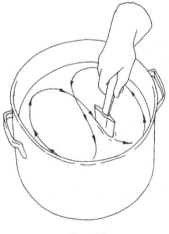

Step 10

Step 11: Incorporate desired nutrients and essential oils to scent the soap, stirring swiftly and thoroughly with the spatula, without beating the mixture.

Step 12: Once the oils are evenly distributed and the soap mixture is uniform in appearance, quickly pour the soap into the frame, moving from one end of the frame to the other to evenly distribute the soap within the frame for uniform bars. Don't scrape any residue from the sides of the pan.

Step 13: Cover the filled soap frame with another empty frame (or a piece of plywood or heavy cardboard); cover with a blanket or two. Leave undisturbed for eighteen to twenty-four hours.

Step 14: Using rulers and a paring knife, lightly mark lines for cutting the mass into bars (do not cut all the way through). Once you are satisfied the lines are straight and uniform, cut through lengthwise and crosswise to the bottom of the frame.

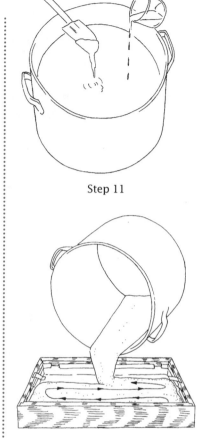

Step 11

Step 12

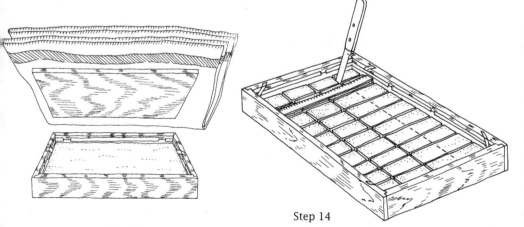

Step 13

Step 14

Step 15: Carefully peel the bars from the paper. Slice a thin sliver off the top of each to remove the powdery white soda ash, and trim any uneven edges.

Step 16: Lay the bars in a single layer on plain brown paper grocery bags, or wicker or rattan placemats.

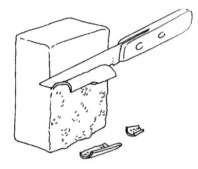

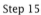

Step 15

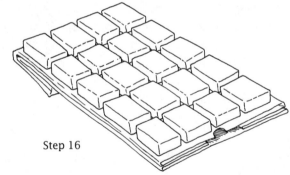

Step 16

SOAP ESSENTIALS BAR
Makes approximately 40 (4-ounce) bars

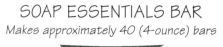

This is the bar my customers request most often. Olive oil is the primary oil used, leaving the soap with a moisturizing sheen once introduced to water. The coconut oil offers a gentle, non-foamy lather and the palm oil makes the bars hard. As you bathe, take the time to flip the bar through your hands a few times to feel the oils and the silky texture. It's quite a contrast to the rough synthetic texture of so many industrially prepared soaps.

This soap combines the very best of soapmaking attributes offered by vegetable oils at an affordable cost. Add your favorite nutrients for even greater skin-care benefit, if desired (see Chapter 6, "Nutrients").

3 pounds cold distilled water (does not need to be refrigerated)
473 grams sodium hydroxide
4 pounds (1.81 kg) olive oil
2 pounds 8 ounces (1.13 kg) coconut oil
1 pound 8 ounces (680 g) palm oil
30 grams grapefruit seed extract (natural preservative), optional
45–50 grams (approximately 15–18 teaspoons) pure essential oil
   (see Chapter 4), optional
Extra nutrients (see Chapter 6), optional

PREPARING YOUR WORK AREA
1. Before beginning, read Chapter 8 and set up your work area and required equipment.
2. Line your mold — a wooden tray or heavy cardboard box (see page 78) — with heavy-duty waxed freezer paper. Be sure to mitre the corners and flatten the paper against the sides of the box. Use masking tape to secure the paper to the box without waves and wrinkles.
3. Measure out the essential oil, preservative, and extra nutrients, and set aside in tightly sealed containers.

MIXING THE KEY INGREDIENTS
4. Put on goggles and gloves. Weigh out the sodium hydroxide and set aside.

5. Set the glass container on the scale and add the distilled water; remove from scale. Carefully add the sodium hydroxide while stirring briskly with a rubber spatula. The fumes will overwhelm you after about ten seconds, so hold your breath while stirring, then leave the room for fresh air. Return after two to three minutes to finish dissolving the sodium hydroxide.

The reaction will heat the lye solution to over 200°F (94°C), so set the bowl aside in a safe place to cool down to 80°F (27°C). If you plan to cool the lye overnight, cover the container tightly to avoid a weakened solution.

6. While the lye is cooling, you can begin mixing the oils. Set the soapmaking pan on the scale and add the olive oil. Then set the 3-quart saucepan on the scale and add the coconut and palm oils. Place pan with the coconut and the palm oils over low heat until most of the solid pieces have melted. The few remaining chunks will melt from the heat in the pan. Pour the heated oils into the olive oil. Should you choose to use a natural preservative, add the grapefruit seed extract to the warm fats and oils, incorporating thoroughly. Let cool to 80°F (27°C).

MAKING THE SOAP

7. You are ready to make soap when the oils and the lye solution have both cooled to 80°F (27°C). If you have cooled the lye overnight and the temperature drops below this point, heat it up by setting the container in a sinkful of hot water. Oils can be heated over low heat on the stove for a short time, if necessary. Remove the pan from the stove once the oils reach 76°F (24°C); the heat in the pan will raise it to 80°F (27°C).

8. Wearing goggles and gloves, slowly drizzle the lye into the oils, stirring briskly as you pour. Continue to stir, circling the edges of the pan and cutting through the middle of the pan to keep as much of the solution as possible in constant motion. Do not beat or whip the mixture, but stir briskly throughout the entire soapmaking process. Do not scrape any residue off the sides of the pan. Once a small amount of soap drizzled across the solution's surface leaves a faint pattern before sinking back into the mass, the soap is ready for the essential oils and nutrients, if desired. This may be from seven to forty minutes, depending upon the variety of olive oil used. (See page 22.) Do not wait until the soap is thick enough for a pattern to remain on the surface, or the soap will harden too quickly once the essential oils are added; yet, be sure that all oils on the surface have been incorporated, leaving a uniform mixture.

9. Incorporate any desired nutrients, and then immediately drizzle in the essential oils to scent the soap, stirring swiftly and thoroughly with a spatula without beating. Stir for twenty to thirty seconds, or as little time as needed to fully incorporate the essential oils. Too much stirring causes streaking and seizing (a quick setup which makes it hard if not impossible to pour the soap into the frames). Pure essential oils are usually more cooperative. Synthetic fragrance oils are more likely to streak and seize.

POURING INTO THE MOLD
10. Once the oils are evenly distributed, quickly pour the soap into the frame without scraping the residue off the sides of the pan. The mixture should be smooth, with no lumps and uniform texture and color. Watery or oily puddles signal a poorly mixed solution that will result in pockets of solid lye in the final bars. Try to pour evenly from one end of the frame to the other for uniform bars. If you see a change in texture, stop pouring.

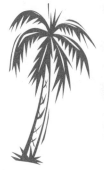

If the last bit of soap mixture at the bottom of the pan is watery and uneven, the stirring process was not quite complete. Do not pollute the rest of your batch by adding this unsaponified portion.

If your first attempt at pouring into the mold is not quick enough and the mixture begins to set unevenly, use a spatula to spread it out to the corners. Keep in mind that the soaps can be trimmed smoothly once the bars are ready to be cut. When this recipe is followed carefully, it is unlikely you will encounter this problem.

CURING AND CUTTING THE BARS
11. Cover the filled frame with another frame, a piece of plywood, or a piece of heavy cardboard; cover with a blanket or

two. Leave undisturbed for eighteen to twenty-four hours. This period is critical, as the insulation allows the soap to heat up and complete the soapmaking process.

12. Uncover the frame and set away from drafts and cold temperatures for one to seven days, or until the soaps are firm enough to cut. Do not wait until they are rock hard.

13. Using rulers and a paring knife, lightly mark the mass into bars, being careful not to cut through. Once the bar marks look straight and uniform, cut lengthwise and cross-wise through to the bottom of the frame. Holding the sides of the waxed paper, lift the entire layer of soaps out of the frame. Carefully peel the bars from the paper, then slice a thin sliver off of the top of each one to remove the powdery white soda ash.* Also trim away any uneven edges.

14. Lay the soaps, in a single layer, on plain brown paper grocery bags, or wicker or rattan placemats. Do not use bags imprinted with ink, as the bars are still alkaline and will pick up the dye. Set the soaps in a dry, well ventilated room, protected from temperature extremes.

15. Allow the soaps to cure for four to six weeks, turning them over once to fully expose the other sides. This is an important period, as the soaps become harder and milder. Wrap as you'd like, preferably in a breathable material.

When sodium hydroxide is exposed to the air, it absorbs water and carbon dioxide to form sodium carbonate, $NaCO_3$. This grayish white powder settles on the top of the soaps as they cure and should be sliced off while trimming the bars. It is not as harsh as sodium hydroxide, but it is drying and irritating to the skin.

VEGETABLE SHAMPOO BAR
for normal to oily hair
Makes approximately 40 (4-ounce) bars

Synthetics have intruded upon all areas of our lives — we need only to read the back of our shampoo bottle for an example. We've learned to carefully examine the list of ingredients on food packages, and yet we don't apply the same scrutiny to personal care products, which are also absorbed into our bodies' systems.

This shampoo bar is solid and can replace liquid shampoo and conditioners. The castor and coconut oils make a rich, thick lather, and the other oils and nutrients clean and condition the hair and scalp.

To use, rub the shampoo bar back and forth across the top of the head to work up a nice lather, then distribute the shampoo throughout the hair. Choose a special soap dish for your shampoo bar to distinguish it from body soaps, even though this bar could certainly be used to clean the body as well.

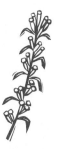

3 pounds (1.36 kg) cold, distilled water (does not need to be refrigerated)
510 grams sodium hydroxide
2 pounds 13 ounces (1.28 kg) olive oil
2 pounds 4 ounces (1.02 kg) castor oil
4 ounces (113 g) jojoba oil
2 pounds 4 ounces (1.02 kg) coconut oil
2 ounces (57 g) each of the following nutrients (optional*): shea butter, sweet almond oil, apricot kernel oil, avocado oil
30 grams grapefruit seed extract (natural preservative), optional
Extra nutrients (added toward the end of the soapmaking process — see Chapter 6), optional
45–50 grams (approximately 15–18 teaspoons) pure essential oil (see Chapter 4), optional

*If you are not using these nutrients, increase the 4 ounces of jojoba oil to 8 ounces, and the amount of olive oil to 3 pounds 1 ounce.

Note: This formula calls for more sodium hydroxide than the SAP value charts suggest. See Chapter 2, Castor Oil, for a detailed explanation.

PREPARING THE WORK AREA
1. Before beginning, read Chapter 8 and set up your work area and required equipment.

2. Line your mold — a wooden tray or heavy cardboard box (see page 78) — with heavy-duty waxed freezer paper. Be sure to mitre the corners and flatten the paper against the sides of the box. Use masking tape to secure the paper to the box without waves and wrinkles.

3. Measure out the essential oil, preservative, and extra nutrients, and set aside in separate tightly sealed containers.

MIXING THE KEY INGREDIENTS

4. Put on goggles and gloves. Weigh out the sodium hydroxide and set aside.

5. Set the 2-quart glass container on the scale and add the distilled water; remove from scale. Carefully add the sodium hydroxide while stirring constantly and briskly with a rubber spatula. The fumes will overwhelm you after about ten seconds, so hold your breath while stirring, and then leave the room for fresh air. Return after two to three minutes to finish dissolving the sodium hydroxide. The reaction will heat the lye solution to over 200°F (93°C); set the bowl aside in a safe place to cool down to 80°F (27°C).

6. While the sodium hydroxide solution is cooling, begin to mix the oils.

Set the soapmaking pan on the scale and add the olive oil, castor oil, jojoba oil, sweet almond oil, apricot kernel oil, and avocado oil. Set the 3-quart saucepan on the scale and add the coconut oil. Place saucepan over low heat until most of the solid pieces of coconut oil are melted. The few remaining chunks will melt from the heat in the pan. Take the saucepan off of the heat and add the shea butter to the melted coconut oil. As you stir, the heated oils will melt the shea butter. Pour the heated coconut oil mixture into the olive oil mixture. Should you choose to use a natural preservative, add

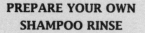

PREPARE YOUR OWN SHAMPOO RINSE

Any shampoo will eventually leave a residue build-up in the hair. Prepare a hair rinse using 1 part apple cider vinegar or lemon juice to 1 part water boiled and cooled. Add 15 to 25 drops of pure essential oil. Store in a spray bottle. Spray on hair after shampooing and rinsing well. Distribute well through the hair and scalp, then quickly rinse well with water.

grapefruit seed extract to the warm fats and oils, incorporating thoroughly.

MAKING THE SHAMPOO BARS

7. Once the lye is falling close to the 80˚F (27˚C) mark, check the temperature of the oils. If the lye temperature falls below 80˚F (27˚C), heat it by setting the container in a sinkful of hot water. To reheat oils dropping below 80˚F (27˚C), place on the stove over low heat for a short time. Remove pan when the temperature reaches 76˚F (24˚C); the heat in the pan will raise temperature to 80˚F (27˚C).

8. With both solutions at 80˚F (27˚C), wearing goggles and gloves, slowly drizzle the lye into the oils, stirring briskly as you pour. Continue to stir, circling the pan and cutting through the middle of the pan to keep as much of the solution as possible in constant motion. Do not beat or whip the mixture, but stir briskly throughout the entire soapmaking process. Do not scrape off any residue from the sides of the pan into the solution.

Depending upon the type of olive oil used (see page 22) the shampoo bars should "trace" within ten to forty minutes. Tracing is when a small amount of the mixture drizzled across the surface leaves a trace of its pattern before sinking back into the mass. Don't wait for the shampoo mixture to be thick enough for the pattern to remain, or the mixture may set up too quickly when the scent is added; yet, be sure that all oils on the surface have been incorporated, leaving a uniform mixture.

9. Incorporate any desired nutrients, and then immediately drizzle in the essential oils, stirring swiftly and thoroughly with the spatula, without beating the mixture. The shampoo bar mixture will incorporate synthetic fragrances better than other soap, but pure essential oils are always a superior choice.

POURING INTO THE MOLD

10. Once the oils are distributed evenly and the mixture is uniform in appearance, quickly pour it into the frame; avoid scraping the residue off the sides of the pan. The mixture should be smooth, with no lumps and uniform texture and color. Try to pour from one end of the frame to the other to distribute the shampoo mixture evenly for uniform bars. Watery or oily puddles signal a poorly mixed solution and will result in pockets of solid lye in the final bars. If you see a change in texture, stop pouring.

If the last bit of mixture at the bottom of the pan is watery and not uniform, do not pollute the rest of your batch by adding this unsaponified portion.

If your first attempt at pouring into the mold is not quick enough, and the mixture begins to set unevenly, use a spatula to spread it out to the corners. Keep in mind that the shampoo bars can be trimmed smoothly once they are ready for cutting. If you follow this recipe carefully, you're unlikely to encounter these troubles.

CURING AND CUTTING THE BARS

11. Cover the filled frame with another empty frame, a piece of plywood, or a piece of heavy cardboard; cover with a blanket or two. Leave undisturbed for eighteen to twenty-four hours. This insulation period is critical, allowing the bars to heat up and complete the process.

12. Uncover the frame and test the mass for firmness. These shampoo bars may be ready to cut soon after opening, for they harden very quickly, unless large quantities of citrus oils have been incorporated. If the bars are still soft, wait until they are firm to cut them into bars. First use a ruler and a paring knife to outline the lines for the bars, then, once satisfied with the look, slice all the way through to the bottom, lengthwise and across.

13. Holding the sides of the waxed paper, lift the mass of shampoo bars out of the frame. Carefully peel each bar from the paper, then slice a thin sliver off of the top to remove the powdery white soda ash. (Shampoo bars will not have as much soda ash as the other soaps.) Trim any uneven edges. Lay the bars in a single layer on plain brown paper grocery bags or wicker or rattan placemats. Do not use bags with ink, as the still-alkaline bars will pick up the dye.

14. Set in a dry, well ventilated room; do not expose to temperature extremes. Allow the shampoo bars to cure for four to six weeks, turning them over once to fully expose the other side. They will harden and become mild during this period. Wrap as you'd like, preferably in a breathable material.

TROPICAL SHAMPOO BAR
for normal to dry hair
Makes approximately 40 (4-ounce) bars

This is my favorite shampoo bar. Less castor oil makes the soapmaking mixture less temperamental, and the bar itself is mild and moisturizing. Though more costly to make than the regular shampoo bar, this formula incorporates sweet almond oil and kukui nut oil, which are wonderful nutrients for the hair and scalp.

3 pounds cold, distilled water (does not need to be refrigerated)
500 grams sodium hydroxide
2 pounds (907 g) olive oil
1 pound 8 ounces (680 g) castor oil
8 ounces (227 g) sweet almond oil
4 ounces (113 g) jojoba oil
4 ounces (113 g) kukui nut oil
2 pounds (907 g) coconut oil
1 pound 8 ounces (680 g) palm oil
30 grams grapefruit seed extract (natural preservative), optional
Extra nutrients (see Chapter 6), optional
45–50 grams (approximately 15–18 teaspoons) pure essential oil
   (see Chapter 4), optional

Note: *This formula calls for more sodium hydroxide than the SAP value charts suggest. See Chapter 2, Castor Oil, for a detailed explanation.*

PREPARING THE WORK AREA
1. Before beginning read Chapter 8 and set up your work area and equipment.

2. Line your mold — a wooden tray or heavy cardboard box (see page 78 for dimensions) — with heavy-duty waxed freezer paper. Be sure to mitre the corners and flatten the paper against the sides of the box. Use masking tape to secure the paper to the box without waves and wrinkles.

3. Measure out the essential oil, preservative, and extra nutrients; set aside in separate tightly sealed containers.

MIXING THE KEY INGREDIENTS

4. Put on goggles and gloves. Weigh out the sodium hydroxide and set aside.

5. Set the 2-quart glass container on the scale and add the distilled water; remove from scale. Carefully add the sodium hydroxide while stirring briskly with a rubber spatula. The fumes will overwhelm you after about ten seconds, so hold your breath while stirring, and then leave the room for fresh air. Return after two to three minutes to finish dissolving the sodium hydroxide. The reaction will heat the lye solution to over 200°F (93°C), so set the bowl aside in a safe place to cool down to 80°F (27°C).

6. While the sodium hydroxide mixture is cooling, begin mixing the oils. Set the soap pan on the scale and add the castor oil, sweet almond oil, jojoba oil, kukui nut oil, and olive oil. Then set the 3-quart saucepan on the scale and add the coconut and palm oils. Place saucepan over low heat until most of the pieces of coconut and palm oils have melted. The few remaining chunks will melt from the heat in the pan. Pour the heated oils into the soapmaking pan with the olive oil mixture. Should you choose to use a natural preservative, add grapefruit seed extract to the warm fats and oils, incorporating thoroughly. Set aside and allow the oils to cool to 80°F (27°C).

MAKING THE SHAMPOO BARS

7. Once both solutions have reached 80°F (27°C) the soapmaking process can proceed. If you cool the lye overnight and the temperature drops below this, it can be reheated over low heat on a stove for a short period. Remove the pan from the stove when it reaches 76°F (24°C); the heat in the pan will raise the temperature to 80°F (27°C). Wearing goggles and gloves, slowly drizzle the lye into the oils, stirring briskly as you pour. Continue to stir, circling the pan and cutting through the middle to keep as much of the solution as possible in constant motion. Do not beat or whip the mixture, but stir briskly throughout the process. Don't scrape off any residue from the sides of the pan into the solution.

Depending upon the type of olive oil used (see page 22) these shampoo bars should "trace" after ten to forty minutes. Tracing occurs when a small amount of the mixture drizzled across the surface leaves a trace of its pattern before sinking back into the mass. If oily puddles still cover the surface, continue stirring until they have been incorporated, leaving a uniform mixture.

8. Mix in any desired nutrients, and then immediately drizzle in the essential oils, stirring swiftly and thoroughly with the spatula, without beating the mixture. The shampoo bars will incorporate synthetic fragrances better than the soaps, but pure essential oils are always a superior choice.

POURING INTO THE MOLD

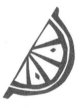

9. Once the oils are distributed evenly and the mixture appears uniform, quickly pour it into the frame without scraping the residue off the sides of the pan. The mixture should be smooth, with no lumps and uniform texture and color. Watery or oily puddles signal a poorly mixed solution and will result in pockets of solid lye within the final bars. Try to pour from one end of the frame to the other to evenly distribute the shampoo mixture within the frame for uniform bars. If you see a change in texture, stop pouring.

If the last bit of mixture at the bottom of the pan is watery and not uniform, do not pollute the rest of your batch by adding this unsaponified portion.

If your first attempt at pouring into the molds is not quick enough, and the mixture begins to set unevenly, use a spatula to spread it out to the corners. Keep in mind that the shampoo bars can be trimmed smoothly once they are ready to be cut. If you follow this recipe carefully, it's unlikely you'll encounter these troubles.

CURING AND CUTTING THE BARS

10. Cover the filled frame with another empty frame, a piece of plywood, or a piece of heavy cardboard; cover with a blanket or two. Leave undisturbed for eighteen to twenty-four hours. This insulation period is critical, allowing the bars to heat up and complete the process.

11. Uncover the frame and test the mass for firmness. These shampoo bars may require up to five to seven days to be sufficiently firm for cutting.

12. Once firm, cut into bars. First use a ruler and a paring knife to outline the bars, then once satisfied with the look, slice all the way through to the bottom, lengthwise and across. Holding the sides of the waxed paper, lift the mass of shampoo bars out of the frame. Carefully, peel the bars from the paper, then slice a thin sliver off of the top of each bar to remove the powdery white soda ash. (Shampoo bars will not have as much soda ash as the other soaps.) Also trim any uneven edges. Lay the bars, single-layer, on plain brown paper grocery bags or wicker or rattan placemats. Do not use bags with ink, as the still alkaline bars will pick up the dye. Set the bags in a dry, well-ventilated room, and do not expose the bars to temperature extremes.

13. Allow the shampoo bars to cure for four to six weeks, turning them over once to fully expose the other sides. They become hard and mild during this period. Wrap as you'd like, preferably in a breathable material.

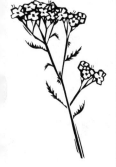

ONE-STOP SOAP
Makes approximately 40 (4-ounce) bars

I call this One-Stop Soap because all the ingredients can be bought in just one trip to a large supermarket. For a beginner who just wants to get started, without committing to many pounds of product, and without putting effort into tracking down ingredients, this recipe is just right. I made just this kind of bar for months in my early soapmaking days. Do keep in mind though, that you pay much higher prices per pound for ingredients bought in supermarket quantities.

One-Stop Soap, like the Soap Essentials Bar, is moisturizing, with that same silky feel. With lots of coconut oil and olive oil, it lathers beautifully and leaves the skin feeling smooth.

Be aware that these bars do not stay as hard as the Soap Essentials Bars do when introduced to water. Vegetable shortening makes a softer bar. This does not mean that the final bars will be soft. It simply means that the bars will take a few weeks longer to harden as they cure, and that once nice and hard, they should not be exposed to an excess of water. They will remain firm if the user keeps the bar away from the constant stream of the shower and places it in a protected soap dish after use. The soap will only get mushy if it goes undiscovered at the bottom of the bathtub for many minutes. Even if this happens, let it spend some time recuperating and hardening back up in the soapdish.

3 pounds (1.36 kg) cold, distilled water (does not need to be refrigerated)
469 7/10 grams sodium hydroxide
3 pounds 8 ounces (1.59 kg) olive oil
2 pounds 8 ounces (1.13 kg) coconut oil
2 pounds (907 g) vegetable shortening
30 grams grapefruit seed extract (natural preservative), optional
Extra nutrients (see Chapter 6), optional
45–50 grams (approximately 15–18 teaspoons) pure essential oil (see Chapter 4), optional

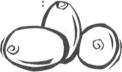

PREPARING THE WORK AREA

1. Before beginning, read Chapter 8 and set up your work area and equipment.

2. Line your mold — a wooden tray or heavy cardboard box (see page 78 for dimensions) — with heavy-duty waxed freezer paper. Be sure to mitre the corners and flatten the paper against the sides of the box. Use masking tape to secure the paper to the box without waves and wrinkles.

3. Measure out the essential oil, preservative, and extra nutrients, and set aside in separate sealed containers.

MIXING THE KEY INGREDIENTS

4. Put on goggles and gloves. Weigh out the sodium hydroxide and set aside.

5. Set the 2-quart glass container on the scale and add the distilled water; remove from scale. Carefully add the sodium hydroxide while stirring briskly with a rubber spatula. The fumes will overwhelm you after about ten seconds, so hold your breath while stirring, and then leave the room for fresh air. Return after two to three minutes to finish dissolving the sodium hydroxide. The reaction will heat the lye solution to over 200°F (93°C), so set the bowl aside in a safe place to cool down to 80°F (27°C). If you plan to cool the lye overnight, cover the container tightly to avoid a weakened solution.

6. While the sodium hydroxide is cooling, begin mixing the oils. Set the soapmaking pan on the scale and add the olive oil. Then set the 3-quart saucepan on the scale and add the coconut oil and the vegetable shortening. Place saucepan over low heat until most of the solid pieces have melted. The few remaining chunks will melt from the heat in the pan. Pour the heated oils into the olive oil. Should you choose to use a natural preservative, add grapefruit seed extract to the warm fats and oils, mixing thoroughly. Let the oils cool to 80°F (27°C).

MAKING THE SOAP

7. You are ready to make soap when the oils and the lye solution both reach 80°F (27°C). If you have cooled the lye overnight and it drops below the desired temperature, heat up the lye by setting the container in a sinkful of hot water. Oils can be reheated over low heat on the stove for a short time. Remove from the stove once the temperature reaches 76°F (24°C); the heat in the pan will raise it to 80°F (27°C).

8. Wearing goggles and gloves, slowly drizzle the lye into the oils, stirring briskly as you pour. Continue to stir, circling the pan and cutting through the middle of the pan to keep as much of the solution as possible in constant motion. Do not beat or whip the mixture, but stir briskly throughout the process. Do not scrape any residue off the sides of the pan. This soap should be ready for essential oils within seven to forty minutes, depending on the variety of olive oil used. (Read about olive oil on page 22.)

Once a small amount of soap can be drizzled across the surface, leaving a trace of that pattern before sinking back into the mass, the soap is ready. Do not wait until the soap is thick enough for a trace to remain on the surface, or the soap will harden too quickly once the essential oils are added; yet, be sure that all oils on the surface have been incorporated, leaving a uniform mixture.

9. Incorporate any desired nutrients, and then immediately drizzle in the essential oils to scent the soaps, stirring swiftly and thoroughly with the spatula, without beating the mixture. Stir for 20 to 30 seconds, or for as little time as needed to fully incorporate the essential oils. Too much stirring causes streaking and seizing (a quick setup which makes it hard if not impossible to pour the soap into the frames). Use pure essential oils for a uniform incorporation of product; synthetic fragrance oils are more likely to streak and seize.

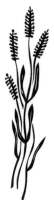

POURING INTO THE MOLD

10. Once the oils are distributed evenly and the soap mixture is uniform in appearance, quickly pour the soap into the frame without scraping the residue off the sides of the pan. Watery or oily puddles signal a poorly mixed solution and will result in pockets of solid lye within the final bars. The mixture should be smooth, with no lumps and uniform texture and color. Try to pour from one end of the frame to the other to evenly distribute the soap within the frame for uniform bars. Stop pouring, should you see a change in texture.

If the last bit of soap mixture at the bottom of the pan is watery and not uniform, the stirring process was not quite complete. Do not pollute the rest of your batch by adding this unsaponified portion. Better to leave it out.

If your first attempt at pouring into the molds is not quick enough, and the mixture begins to set unevenly, use a spatula to spread it out to the corners. Keep in mind that the soaps can be trimmed smoothly once the bars are ready to be cut. When this recipe is carefully followed, it is unlikely that you will encounter these troubles. Cover the frame with another frame, a piece of plywood, or a piece of heavy cardboard, then finally with a blanket or two. Leave undisturbed for eighteen to twenty-four hours. This period is critical, as the insulation allows the soap to heat up and complete the soapmaking process.

CURING AND CUTTING THE BARS

11. Uncover the frame and set away from drafts and cold temperatures for one to seven days, or until the soaps are firm enough to cut. Do not wait until they are rock hard.

12. Using rulers and a paring knife, lightly (do not cut all the way through) mark the mass into bars. Once the bars seem straight and uniform, cut lengthwise and crosswise through to the bottom of the frame. Holding the sides of the waxed paper, lift the soaps out of the frame. Carefully peel the soaps from the paper, then slice a thin sliver off of the top of each bar to remove the powdery white soda ash (see asterisk following the Soap Essentials Bar recipe). Also trim any uneven edges.

13. Lay the soaps, in a single layer, on plain brown paper grocery bags, or wicker or rattan placemats. Do not use bags imprinted with ink, as the bars are still alkaline and will pick up the dye. Set the bags in a dry, well ventilated room, and do not expose the soaps to temperature extremes.

14. Allow the soaps to continue to cure for four to six weeks, turning them over once to fully expose the other sides. This is an important period, as the soaps become harder and more mild. Wrap as you'd like, preferably in a breathable material.

GOURMET BAR
Makes approximately 40 (4-ounce) bars

These are the "sterling" of soap bars, packed with some of the most effective nutrients and oils known to soapmaking. The ingredients are expensive, so I consider Gourmet Bars more of an indulgence than part of a routine. But for those friends or strangers you'd like to spoil once in a while, here is a suggestion. Do save a few bars for yourself.

These must be experienced to appreciate.

3 pounds cold, distilled water (does not need to be refrigerated)
475 grams sodium hydroxide
2 pounds (907 g) olive oil
½ pound (227 g) sweet almond oil
½ pound (227 g) apricot kernel oil
½ pound (227 g) kukui nut oil
½ pound (227 g) jojoba oil
2 pounds 8 ounces (1.13 kg) coconut oil
1 pound 8 ounces (680 g) palm oil
4 ounces (113 g) shea butter (also known as African karite butter)
30 grams grapefruit seed extract (natural preservative), optional
Extra nutrients (see Chapter 6), optional
45–50 grams (approximately 15–18 teaspoons) pure essential oil
   (see Chapter 4), optional

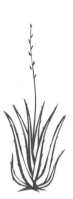

PREPARING THE WORK AREA

1. Before beginning, read Chapter 8 and set up your work area and equipment.

2. Line your mold — a wooden tray or heavy cardboard box (see page 78 for dimensions) — with heavy-duty waxed freezer paper. Be sure to mitre the corners and flatten the paper against the sides of the box. Use masking tape to secure the paper to the box without waves and wrinkles.

3. Measure out the essential oil, preservative, and extra nutrients, and set aside in separate tightly sealed containers.

MIXING THE KEY INGREDIENTS

4. Put on goggles and gloves. Weigh out the sodium hydroxide and set aside.

5. Set the 2-quart glass container on the scale and add the distilled water; remove from scale. Carefully add the sodium hydroxide while stirring briskly with a rubber spatula. The fumes will overwhelm you after about ten seconds, so hold your breath while stirring, and then leave the room for fresh air. Return after two to three minutes to finish dissolving the sodium hydroxide. The reaction will heat the lye solution to over 200°F (93°C), so set the bowl aside in a safe place to cool down to 80°F (27°C). If you plan to cool the lye overnight, cover the container tightly to avoid a weakened solution.

6. While the sodium hydroxide mixture is cooling, begin

mixing the oils. Set the soapmaking pan on the scale and add the olive oil, sweet almond oil, apricot kernel oil, kukui nut oil, and jojoba oil. Then set the 3-quart saucepan on the scale and add the coconut oil, palm oil, and shea butter. Place saucepan over low heat until most of the solid pieces have melted. The few remaining chunks will melt from the heat within the pan. Pour the heated oils into the olive oil mixture. Should you choose to use a natural preservative, add grape-fruit seed extract to the warm fats and oils, mixing thorough-ly. Let the oils cool to 80°F (27°C).

MAKING THE SOAP

7. You are ready to make soap when the oils and the lye solution both reach 80°F (27°C). If you have cooled the lye overnight and the temperature drops below the desired degrees, heat up the lye by setting the container in a sinkful of hot water. Oils can be reheated over low heat on the stove for a short time. Remove pan from heat when temperature reaches 76°F (24°C); heat in pan will raise it to 80°F (27°C).

8. Wearing goggles and gloves, slowly drizzle the lye into the oils, stirring briskly as you pour. Continue to stir, cir-cling the pan and cutting through the middle of the pan to keep as much of the solution as possible in constant motion. Do not beat or whip the mixture, but stir briskly throughout the process. Don't scrape any residue off the sides of the pan. This soap should be ready for essential oils within seven to forty minutes.

Once a small amount of soap can be drizzled across the surface, leaving a trace of that pattern before sinking back into the mass, the soap is ready. Do not wait until the soap is thick enough for a trace to remain on the surface, or the soap will harden too quickly once the essential oils are added; yet, be sure that all oils on the surface have been incorporated, leaving a uniform mixture.

9. Incorporate any desired nutrients, and then immediate-ly drizzle in the essential oils to scent the soaps, stirring swiftly and thoroughly with the spatula, without beating the mixture. Stir for twenty to thirty seconds, or for as little time as needed to fully incorporate the essential oils. Too much stirring causes streaking and seizing (a quick setup which makes it hard if not impossible to pour the soap into the frames). Use pure essential oils to scent these gourmet bars. The ingredients are far too costly and pure to pollute the batch with a final splash of synthetic fragrance.

POURING INTO THE MOLD

10. Once the oils are evenly distributed and the soap mixture is uniform in appearance, quickly pour the soap into the frame without scraping the residue off the sides of the pan. Watery or oily puddles signal a poorly mixed solution and will result in pockets of solid lye within the final bars. The mixture should be smooth, with no lumps and uniform texture and color. Try to pour from one end of the frame to the other to evenly distribute the soap within the frame for uniform bars. Stop pouring, should you see a change in texture.

If the last bit of soap mixture at the bottom of the pan is watery and not uniform, the stirring process was not quite complete. Do not pollute the rest of your batch by adding this unsaponified portion. Better to leave it out.

If your first attempt is not quick enough, and the mixture begins to set unevenly, use a spatula to spread it out to the corners. Keep in mind that the soaps can be trimmed smoothly once the bars are ready to be cut. Cover the frame with another frame, a piece of plywood, or a piece of heavy cardboard, then finally with a blanket or two. Leave undisturbed for eighteen to twenty-four hours. This period is critical, as the insulation allows the soap to heat up and complete the soapmaking process.

CURING AND CUTTING THE BARS

11. Uncover the frame and set away from drafts and cold temperatures for one to seven days, or until the soaps are firm enough to cut. Do not wait until they are rock hard.

12. Using rulers and a paring knife, lightly (do not cut all the way through) mark the mass into bars. Once the bars seem straight and uniform, cut lengthwise and crosswise through to the bottom of the frame. Holding the sides of the waxed paper, lift the soaps out of the frame. Carefully peel the soaps from the paper, then slice a thin sliver off of the top of each bar to remove the powdery white soda ash (see asterisk following the Soap Essentials Bar recipe on page 94). Also trim any uneven edges.

13. Lay the soaps, in a single layer, on plain brown paper grocery bags, or wicker or rattan placemats. Do not use bags imprinted with ink, as the bars are still alkaline and will pick up the dye. Set the bags in a dry, well ventilated room, and do not expose the soaps to temperature extremes.

14. Allow the soaps to continue to cure for four to six weeks, turning them over once to fully expose the other sides. This is an important period, as the soaps become harder and more mild. Wrap as you'd like, preferably in a breathable material.

GOAT MILK SOAP
Makes approximately 40 (4-ounce) bars

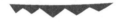

This bar offers all of the qualities of the Soap Essentials Bar, plus the extra moisturizing quality of goat milk. I add only enough goat milk to affect the blend, for too much makes the soap more vulnerable to premature rancidity.

Though the inclusion of goat milk involves a bit more precision and fussing, it is fun to experiment with other recipes. I love to scent these bars with one of the sassafras blends. This soap is homey and fresh.

2½ pounds (1.13 kg) cold, distilled water (does not need to be refrigerated)
473 grams sodium hydroxide
4 pounds (1.81 kg) olive oil
2 pounds 8 ounces (1.13 kg) coconut oil
1 pound 8 ounces (680 g) palm oil
30 grams grapefruit seed extract (natural preservative), optional

2 ²/₁₀ grams tocopherol (natural preservative), optional
½ pound (227 g) cold goat milk
Extra nutrients (see Chapter 6), optional
45–50 grams (approximately 15–18 teaspoons) pure essential oil
   (see Chapter 4), optional

PREPARING THE WORK AREA
1. Before beginning, read Chapter 8 and set up your work area and equipment.
2. Line your mold — a wooden tray or heavy cardboard box (see page 78 for dimensions) — with heavy-duty waxed freezer paper. Be sure to mitre the corners and flatten the paper against the sides of the box. Use masking tape to secure the paper to the box without waves and wrinkles.
3. Measure out the essential oil, preservatives, and extra nutrients, and set aside in separate tightly sealed containers.

MIXING THE KEY INGREDIENTS
4. Put on goggles and gloves. Weigh out the sodium hydroxide and set aside.
5. Set the 2-quart glass container on the scale and add the distilled water; remove from scale. Carefully add the sodium hydroxide while stirring briskly with a rubber spatula. The fumes will overwhelm you after about ten seconds, so hold your breath while stirring, and then leave the room for fresh air. Return after two to three minutes to finish dissolving the sodium hydroxide. The reaction will heat the lye solution to over 200°F (93°C), so set the bowl aside in a safe place to cool down to 80°F (27°C).

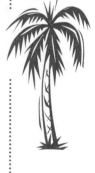

6. While the sodium hydroxide solution cools, begin mixing the oils. Set the soapmaking pan on the scale and add the olive oil. Then set the 3-quart saucepan on the scale and add the coconut and the palm oils. Place saucepan over low heat until most of the solid pieces of the oils have melted. The few remaining chunks will melt from the heat within the pan. Pour the heated oils into the olive oil. Should you choose to use natural preservatives (see chapter 7), add the grapefruit seed extract and the tocopherol to the warm fats and oils, mixing thoroughly. Let the oils cool to 80°F (27°C).

MAKING THE SOAP

7. As the lye solution approaches 80°F (27°C), gently heat the goat milk to 80°F (27°C), stirring gently and constantly. At this time, be sure that the oils are at 80°F (27°C), so the oils will be ready and waiting. If they are too cool, heat the pan over very low heat, removing the pan from the stove when the oils reach 76°F (24°C). (The heat of the oils will bring the solution to the 80°F (27°C) mark.)

8. Now add the lye solution to the goat milk, drizzling the lye in slowly and stirring the mixture briskly to avoid curdling. Combining the lye with the milk may cause the mixture to heat up by a few degrees, though probably no higher than 84° to 85°F (29°C).

9. Wearing goggles and gloves, slowly drizzle the lye/goat milk solution into the oils, stirring briskly as you pour. Continue to stir, circling the pan and cutting through the middle of the pan to keep as much of the solution as possible in constant motion. Do not beat or whip the mixture, but stir 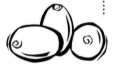 briskly throughout the entire process. Don't scrape any residue off the sides of the pan. This soap may be slightly grainy, and will take anywhere from ten to forty minutes to saponify, depending on the variety of olive oil used and upon how closely the temperatures have been followed. (Read about olive oil on page 22.)

Once a small amount of soap can be drizzled across the surface, leaving a trace of that pattern before sinking back into the mass, the soap is ready for essential oils. And yet, be sure that all oils on the surface have been incorporated, leaving a uniform mixture.

10. Incorporate any desired nutrients, and then immediately drizzle in the essential oils to scent the soaps, stirring swiftly and thoroughly with the spatula, without beating the mixture. Stir for twenty to thirty seconds, or as little time as needed to fully incorporate the essential oils. Too much stirring causes streaking and seizing (a quick setup which makes it hard if not impossible to pour the soap into the frames). Use pure essential oils for a uniform incorporation of product; synthetic fragrance oils are more likely to streak and seize.

POURING INTO THE MOLD

11. Quickly pour the soap into the frame without scraping the residue off the sides of the pan. The mixture should be nice and uniform. Try to pour from one end of the frame to the other to evenly distribute the soap within the frame for uniform bars. If your first attempt is not quick enough, and the mixture begins to set unevenly, use a spatula to spread it out to the corners. Keep in mind that the soaps can be trimmed smoothly once the bars are ready to be cut.

If the last bit of soap mixture at the bottom of the pan is watery and not uniform, the stirring process was not quite complete. Watery or oily puddles signal a poorly mixed solution and will result in pockets of solid lye within the final bars. Do not pollute the rest of your batch by adding this unsaponified portion. Better to leave it out.

CURING AND CUTTING THE BARS

12. Cover the frame with another frame, a piece of plywood, or a piece of heavy cardboard, then finally with a blanket or two. Leave undisturbed for eighteen to twenty-four hours. This period is critical, as the insulation allows the soap to heat up and complete the soapmaking process.

13. Uncover the frame and set away from drafts and cold temperatures for one to seven days, or until the soaps are firm enough to cut. Do not wait until they are rock hard.

14. Using rulers and a paring knife, lightly (do not cut all the way through) mark the mass into bars. Once the bars seem straight and uniform, cut lengthwise and crosswise through to the bottom of the frame. Holding the sides of the waxed paper, lift the soaps out of the frame. Carefully peel the soaps from the paper, then slice a thin sliver off of the top of each bar to remove the powdery white soda ash (see asterisk following the Soap Essentials Bar recipe on page 94). Also trim any uneven edges.

15. Lay the soaps, in a single layer, on plain brown paper grocery bags, or wicker or rattan placemats. Do not use bags imprinted with ink, as the bars are still alkaline and will pick up the dye. Set the bags in a dry, well ventilated room, and do not expose the soaps to temperature extremes.

16. Allow the soaps to continue to cure for four to six weeks, turning them over once to fully expose the other sides. This is an important period, as the soaps become harder and more mild. Wrap as you'd like, preferably in a breathable material.

AVOCADO SOAP
Makes approximately 40 (4-ounce) bars

Resist the temptation to color this soap an artificial shade of green. Avocado oil is a remarkable vegetable oil, one of the most gentle of all. People with sensitive skin usually respond well to this formula. It is superfatted, with some unsaponified avocado oil added just before pouring. Any superfatted soap is more prone to rancidity, but this bar is worth the shorter shelf life. Add the grapefruit seed oil for greater protection.

3 pounds (1.36 kg) cold, distilled water (does not need to be
    refrigerated)
470 $\frac{7}{10}$ grams sodium hydroxide
3 pounds (1.36 kg) avocado oil
1 pound (454 g) olive oil
2 pounds 8 ounces (1.13 kg) coconut oil
1 pound 8 ounces (680 g) palm oil
30 grams grapefruit seed extract (natural preservative), optional
2 tablespoons (30 ml) of additional avocado oil (add just before
    pouring soap into the frame)
Extra nutrients (see Chapter 6), optional
45–50 grams (approximately 15–18 teaspoons) pure essential oil
    (see Chapter 4), optional

PREPARING THE WORK AREA
1. Before beginning, read Chapter 8 and set up your work area and equipment.
2. Line your mold — a wooden tray or heavy cardboard box (see page 78 for dimensions) — with heavy-duty waxed freezer paper. Be sure to mitre the corners and flatten the paper against the sides of the box. Use masking tape to secure the

paper to the box without waves and wrinkles.

3. Measure out the essential oil, preservative, and the extra nutrients (including the 2 additional tablespoons of avocado oil), and set aside in tightly sealed containers.

MIXING THE KEY INGREDIENTS

4. Put on goggles and gloves. Weigh out the sodium hydroxide and set aside.

5. Set the 2-quart glass container on the scale and add the distilled water; remove from scale. Carefully add the sodium hydroxide while stirring briskly with a rubber spatula. The fumes will overwhelm you after about ten seconds, so hold your breath while stirring, and then leave the room for fresh air. Return after two to three minutes to finish dissolving the sodium hydroxide. The reaction will heat the lye solution to over 200°F (93°C), so set the bowl aside in a safe place to cool down to 80°F (27°C). If you plan to cool the lye overnight, cover the container tightly to avoid a weakened solution.

6. While the sodium hydroxide mixture is cooling, begin mixing the oils. Set the soapmaking pan on the scale and add the avocado oil and the olive oil. Then set the 3-quart saucepan on the scale and add the coconut and palm oils. Place saucepan over low heat until most of the solid pieces have melted. The few remaining chunks will melt from the heat within the pan. Pour the heated oils into the olive oil. Should you choose to use a natural preservative, add grapefruit seed extract to the warm fats and oils, incorporating thoroughly. Let the oils cool to 80°F (27°C).

MAKING THE SOAP

7. You are ready to make soap when the oils and the lye solution both reach 80°F (27°C). If you have cooled the lye overnight and the temperature drops below the desired temperature, heat up the lye by setting the container in a sinkful of hot water. Oils can be reheated over low heat on the stove for a short time. Remove from stove once the oil reaches 76°F (24°C); the heat within the pan will raise the temperature to 80°F (27°C).

8. Wearing goggles and gloves, slowly drizzle the lye into the oils, stirring briskly as you pour. Continue to stir, circling the pan and cutting through the middle to keep as much of the solution as possible in constant motion. Do not beat or whip the mixture, but stir briskly throughout the process. Don't scrape any residue off the sides of the pan. This soap should be ready for essential oils within seven to forty minutes, depending on the variety of olive oil used. (Read about olive oil on page 22.)

Once a small amount of soap can be drizzled across the surface, leaving a trace of that pattern before sinking back into the mass, the soap is ready. Do not wait until the soap is thick enough for a trace to remain on the surface, or the soap will harden too quickly once the essential oils are added; yet, be sure that all oils on the surface have been incorporated, leaving a uniform mixture.

9. Gently but thoroughly incorporate the two tablespoons of avocado oil. This extra oil will superfat the mixture further.

10. Immediately drizzle in the essential oils to scent the soap, stirring swiftly and thoroughly with the spatula, without beating the mixture. Stir for twenty to thirty seconds, or for as little time as needed to fully incorporate the essential oils. Too much stirring causes streaking and seizing (a quick setup which makes it hard if not impossible to pour the soap into the frames). Use pure essential oils for a uniform incorporation of product; synthetic fragrance oils are more likely to streak and seize.

POURING INTO THE MOLD
11. Once the oils are evenly distributed and the soap mixture is uniform in appearance, quickly pour the soap into the frame without scraping the residue off the sides of the pan. Watery or oily puddles signal a poorly mixed solution and will result in pockets of solid lye within the final bars. The mixture should be smooth, with no lumps and uniform texture and color. Try to pour from one end of the frame to the other to evenly distribute the soap within the frame for uniform bars. Stop pouring, should you see a change in texture.

If the last bit of soap mixture at the bottom of the pan is watery and not uniform, the stirring process was not quite complete. Do not pollute the rest of your batch by adding this unsaponified portion. Better to leave it out.

If your first attempt at pouring into the molds is not quick enough, and the mixture begins to set unevenly, use a spatula to spread it out to the corners. Keep in mind that the soaps can be trimmed smoothly once the bars are ready to be cut. When this recipe is carefully followed, it is unlikely that you will encounter these troubles. Cover the frame with another frame, a piece of plywood, or a piece of heavy cardboard, then finally with a blanket or two. Leave undisturbed for eighteen to twenty-four hours. This period is critical, as the insulation allows the soap to heat up and complete the soapmaking process.

CURING AND CUTTING THE BARS

12. Uncover the frame and set away from drafts and cold temperatures for one to seven days, or until the soaps are firm enough to cut. Do not wait until they are rock hard.

13. Using rulers and a paring knife, lightly (do not cut all the way through) mark the mass into bars. Once the bars seem straight and uniform, cut lengthwise and crosswise through to the bottom of the frame. Holding the sides of the waxed paper, lift the soaps out of the frame. Carefully peel the soaps from the paper, then slice a thin sliver off of the top of each bar to remove the powdery white soda ash (see asterisk following the Soap Essentials Bar recipe). Also trim any uneven edges.

14. Lay the soaps, in a single layer, on plain brown paper grocery bags, or wicker or rattan placemats. Do not use bags imprinted with ink, as the bars are still alkaline and will pick up the dye. Set the bags in a dry, well ventilated room, and do not expose the soaps to temperature extremes.

15. Allow the soaps to continue to cure for four to six weeks, turning them over once to fully expose the other sides. This is an important period, as the soaps become harder and more mild. Wrap as you'd like, preferably in a breathable material.

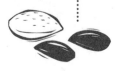

TOUCH OF TALLOW BAR
Makes approximately 40 (4-ounce) bars

For those people who would like to compare vegetable soap to tallow soap, I've included a tallow formula. Of course, most soapmakers would not call this a tallow soap, since it only includes 18.75 percent tallow. But, considering tallow's limitations with respect to skin care, it should only be used with beneficial oils.

I've included lots of olive oil for its moisturizing quality, and the coconut oil offers a nice lather. Avocado and sweet almond oils are gentle and effective nutrients. If necessary, an extra pound of olive oil can be substituted for the other more costly oils.

3 pounds (1.36 kg) cold, distilled water (does not need to be
   refrigerated)
472 grams sodium hydroxide
3 pounds (1.36 kg) olive oil
½ pound (227 g) avocado oil
2 pounds 8 ounces (1.13 kg) coconut oil
1 pound 8 ounces (680 g) rendered tallow
½ pound (227 g) sweet almond oil
30 grams grapefruit seed extract (natural preservative), optional
2 ³⁄₁₀ grams tocopherol (natural preservative), optional
Extra nutrients (see Chapter 6), optional
45–50 grams (approximately 15–18 teaspoons) pure essential oil
   (see Chapter 4), optional

PREPARING THE WORK AREA
1. Before beginning, read Chapter 8 and set up your work area and equipment.
2. Line your mold — a wooden tray or heavy cardboard box (see page 78 for dimensions) — with heavy-duty waxed freezer paper. Be sure to mitre the corners and flatten the paper against the sides of the box. Use masking tape to secure the paper to the box without waves and wrinkles.
3. Measure out the essential oil, preservatives, and extra nutrients and set aside in separate tightly sealed containers.

MIXING THE KEY INGREDIENTS

4. Put on goggles and gloves. Weigh out the sodium hydroxide and set aside.

5. Set the 2-quart glass container on the scale and add the distilled water; remove from scale. Carefully add the sodium hydroxide while stirring briskly with a rubber spatula. The fumes will overwhelm you after about ten seconds, so hold your breath while stirring, and then leave the room for fresh air. Return after two to three minutes to finish dissolving the sodium hydroxide. The reaction will heat the lye solution to over 200°F (93°C), so set the bowl aside in a safe place to cool down to 80°F (27°C). If you plan to cool the lye overnight, cover the container tightly to avoid a weakened solution.

6. While the sodium hydroxide mixture is cooling, begin mixing the oils. Set the soapmaking pan on the scale and add the olive, avocado, and sweet almond oils. Then set the 3-quart saucepan on the scale and add the coconut oil and the tallow. Place saucepan over low heat until most of the solid pieces have melted. The few remaining chunks will melt from the heat within the pan. Pour the heated oils into the olive oil mixture. Should you choose to use natural preservatives, add grapefruit seed extract and tocopherol to the warm fats and oils, mixing thoroughly. Let the oils cool to 80°F (27°C).

MAKING THE SOAP

7. You are ready to make soap when the oils and the lye solution both reach 80°F (27°C). If you have cooled the lye overnight and the temperature drops below the desired temperature, heat up the lye by setting the container in a sinkful of hot water. Oils can be reheated over low heat on the stove for a short time, if necessary. Remove from heat when it reaches 76°F (24°C); the heat in the pan will raise temperature to 80°F (27°C).

8. Wearing goggles and gloves, slowly drizzle the lye into the oils, stirring briskly as you pour. Continue to stir, circling the pan and cutting through the middle to keep as much of the solution as possible in constant motion. Do not beat or whip the mixture, but stir briskly throughout the process. Don't scrape any residue off the sides of the pan. This soap should be ready for essential oils within seven to twenty minutes.

Once a small amount of soap can be drizzled across the surface, leaving a trace of that pattern before sinking back into the mass, the soap is ready. Do not wait until the soap is thick enough for a trace to remain on the surface, or the soap will harden too quickly once the essential oils are added; yet, be sure that all oils on the surface have been incorporated, leaving a uniform mixture.

9. Incorporate any desired nutrients, and then immediately drizzle in the essential oils to scent the soaps, stirring swiftly and thoroughly with the spatula, without beating the mixture. Stir for twenty to thirty seconds, or for as little time as needed to fully incorporate the essential oils. Too much stirring causes streaking and seizing (a quick setup which makes it hard if not impossible to pour the soap into the frames). Use pure essential oils for a uniform incorporation of product; synthetic fragrance oils are more likely to streak and seize.

POURING INTO THE MOLD

10. Once the oils are evenly distributed and the soap mixture is uniform in appearance, quickly pour the soap into the frame without scraping the residue off the sides of the pan. Watery or oily puddles signal a poorly mixed solution and will result in pockets of solid lye within the final bars. The mixture should be smooth, with no lumps and uniform texture and color. Try to pour from one end of the frame to the other to evenly distribute the soap within the frame for uniform bars. Stop pouring, should you see a change in texture.

If the last bit of soap mixture at the bottom of the pan is watery and not uniform, the stirring process was not quite complete. Do not pollute the rest of your batch by adding this unsaponified portion. Better to leave it out.

If your first attempt at pouring into the molds is not quick enough, and the mixture begins to set unevenly, use a spatula to spread it out to the corners. Keep in mind that the soaps can be trimmed smoothly once the bars are ready to be cut. When this recipe is carefully followed, it is unlikely that you will encounter these troubles.

CURING AND CUTTING THE BARS

11. Cover the frame with another frame, a piece of plywood, or a piece of heavy cardboard, then finally with a blanket or two. Leave undisturbed for eighteen to twenty-four hours. This period is critical, as the insulation allows the soap to heat up and complete the soapmaking process.

12. Uncover the frame and set away from drafts and cold temperatures for one to seven days, or until the soaps are firm enough to cut. Do not wait until they are rock hard.

13. Using rulers and a paring knife, lightly (do not cut all the way through) mark the mass into bars. Once the bars seem straight and uniform, cut lengthwise and crosswise through to the bottom of the frame. Holding the sides of the waxed paper, lift the soaps out of the frame. Carefully peel the soaps from the paper, then slice a thin sliver off of the top of each bar to remove the powdery white soda ash (see asterisk following the Soap Essentials Bar recipe on page 94). Also trim any uneven edges.

14. Lay the soaps, in a single layer, on plain brown paper grocery bags, or wicker or rattan placemats. Do not use bags imprinted with ink, as the bars are still alkaline and will pick up the dye. Set the bags in a dry, well ventilated room, and do not expose the soaps to temperature extremes.

15. Allow the soaps to continue to cure for four to six weeks, turning them over once to fully expose the other sides. This is an important period, as the soaps become harder and more mild. Wrap as you'd like, preferably in a breathable material.

MIX AND MATCH RECIPES

Using any of the eight basic soap recipes on pages 91–118 as a foundation, you can design variations by incorporating one or more of the many soapmaking nutrients (see pages 58–67 for more on nutrients). Some nutrients are added at the end of the soapmaking process, but some, like the vitamin oils, are included from the start. For those that are added just before the pure essential oils, be sure that the soap has saponified before proceeding with these final touches.

Note that adding these rich nutrients at the end of the soap-making process makes a superfatted soap. Superfatted soap is mild and moisturizing (my preference!), but is likely to have a shorter shelf life. While testing new formulas, always follow the basic soapmaking instructions carefully.

The following suggestions may help trigger ideas for many other possibilities. Develop oil and nutrient combinations with specific skin-care needs in mind, or with no rhyme or reason. Just be sure to have fun playing with the combinations.

OATMEAL/HONEY SOAP

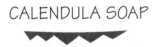

Additions:
½–1 cup (118–237 ml) finely ground oatmeal
4 tablespoons (59 ml) honey, slightly warmed
45 grams (approximately 15 teaspoons) essential oil
    (see Chapter 4), optional

Before beginning, read about incorporating oatmeal and honey in Chapter 6 (page 66).

Use your favorite basic soap recipe. Blend the finely ground oatmeal into the saponified soap mixture, stirring well to avoid clumps. Incorporate the slightly warmed honey into the mixture, and finally add pure essential oil if desired.

CALENDULA SOAP

Additions:
½ cup (118 ml) finely ground calendula flowers
4 tablespoons (59 ml) calendula oil
45 grams (approximately 15 teaspoons) essential oil (see Chapter 4), as desired

Begin preparing your favorite basic soap recipe. Once the soap has saponified, thoroughly incorporate the finely ground calendula flowers; gently blend in the calendula oil. Finally, add essential oil if desired. Replace up to 1 pound of your soap-making oils with calendula oil for greater benefit.

MIXED NUTS BAR

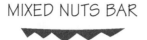

Additions:
5 teaspoons (25 ml) bitter almond oil
10 teaspoons (50 ml) lemon oil
½ cup (118 ml) finely ground almonds
2 tablespoons (30 ml) sweet almond oil
2 tablespoons (30 ml) kukui nut oil

In a small container, combine the bitter almond oil and lemon oil; cover these essential oils and set aside.

Prepare your favorite basic soap recipe. Once the soap has saponified, thoroughly incorporate the finely ground almonds. Gently blend in the sweet almond oil and kukui nut oil. Finally, add the essential oil mixture.

SOUTHWEST SOAP

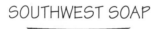

Additions:
5 teaspoons (25 ml) juniper berry oil
4 teaspoons (20 ml) red thyme oil
4 teaspoons (20 ml) lavender oil
2 teaspoons (10 ml) rosemary oil
½ cup (118 ml) cornmeal
4 tablespoons (59 ml) jojoba oil

In a small container, combine the juniper berry oil, red thyme oil, lavender oil, and rosemary oil. Cover these essential oils and set aside.

Prepare your favorite basic soap recipe. Just before pouring the saponified soap into frames, thoroughly blend the

A SOAPMAKER'S STORY
Catherine Failor/Copra Soaps

Catherine Failor says, "The idea for the line of soaps I have now came as an epiphany. I know this might sound hokey, but I was walking through a room of my house, not even thinking about soap — hadn't made any for a couple of years — when in a brilliant flash of color, I had a vision of my patterned soaps. With this vision came the understanding that these soaps would be my business. It was not a conscious thought or decision. It just *was*. Therefore, I never had to agonize or worry over the success or failure of my eventual business because it always had seemed like something that was meant to be."

After a year of "sometimes excruciating trial and error," Catherine perfected the method of casting patterned, all-vegetable soaps. She designed much of the cutting equipment herself, using pneumatic presses to push slabs of soap through differently shaped cutters.

Copra Soaps are striking — each bar looks like a piece of modern art. Some are striped, others are patterned with stars, circles, triangles, and trapezoids. The colors (created with synthetic dyes) are bright and contrasting: red and white on black; jade on purple; yellow on turqoise; alternating stripes of the rainbow.

For two and a half years, Catherine worked out of her basement, but Copra Soaps grew quickly, and she now has a 3,500 square foot shop with four to six people working with her, depending upon the season. The soap is mixed in 100-gallon, stainless steel containers, 700 to 800 pounds at a time. Catherine studied turn-of-the-century soapmaking books and found a design for soap molds which hold around 350 pounds of soap.

Copra Soaps' location is a soapmaker's dream — just a mile from the port of Portland, Oregon, where tankers from Malaysia bring in tropical oils. "It's a great setup," says Catherine. "I bring my empty drums in for refilling and just truck them back to my shop."

Catherine Failor is a reminder to us all to do more than just imitate what we've already seen — to let our soaps reflect a piece of ourselves.

cornmeal into the soap mixture. Then add four tablespoons of jojoba oil, and blend well. Add the pure essential oil mixture immediately.

BORAGE BAR

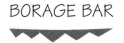

Additions:
2 tablespoons (30 ml) borage oil
2 tablespoons (30 ml) kukui nut oil
45 grams (approximately 15 teaspoons) pure essential oil (see Chapter 4), optional

Prepare your favorite basic soap recipe. Just before pouring the saponified soap into frames, thoroughly incorporate the borage oil and kukui nut oil (you may substitute evening primrose oil for the borage oil). Add pure essential oil if desired. Replace up to 1 pound of your soapmaking oils with borage oil for greater benefit.

VITAMIN SOAP

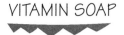

Additions:
2 tablespoons (30 ml) wheat germ oil
2 tablespoons (30 ml) carrot seed oil
2 tablespoons (30 ml) carrot root oil
2 tablespoons (30 ml) vitamin E oil
4 tablespoons (59 ml) avocado oil
45–50 grams (approximately 15–18 teaspoons) pure essential oil (see Chapter 4), optional

Prepare your favorite basic soap recipe. Replace ½ cup of the olive oil with 2 tablespoons each of wheatgerm oil, carrot seed oil, carrot root oil, and vitamin E oil. (You may increase the quantity of one of these oils to substitute for another you don't have on hand.) These vitamin oils are added along with the other soapmaking oils at the beginning of the soapmaking process.

Once the soap has saponified, add the avocado oil and pure essential oil, if desired, blending thoroughly before pouring the soap into frames.

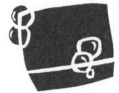

CHAPTER 10
Diagnosing Signs of Trouble

▼▼▼▼

Early in my soapmaking days, another soapmaker encouraged me to take careful notes of each and every soapmaking — the exact amounts of the ingredients used, along with a detailed description of each step in the process. Benefiting from my many failed batches, you can avoid most of the following pitfalls, but careful note-taking will help ensure you don't make the same mistakes twice.

Nearly all of the problems listed here are related to imprecision. You can avoid most of them by following directions carefully, and regularly testing scales and thermometers for accuracy. Remember, as frustrating as the occasional failure is, most mistakes are small, and soap is forgiving. The major goofs are lifetime lessons.

Test the pH of any suspicious bars. Read the instructions on page 131 before taking any action.

DIAGNOSING SIGNS OF TROUBLE WITHIN THE SOAP PAN

Trouble Sign	Reasons Why	What to Do
Mixture in pan not tracing	◆ Not enough lye ◆ Too much water ◆ Incorrect temperatures ◆ Stirring too slowly	Check your measurements to be sure that the correct amounts were used; be sure that you are stirring briskly and consistently. If everything seems to be on track, continue stirring for as long as you can manage, but no longer than four hours. If the mixture separates into oily and watery layers, even after a few hours, give up on the batch. If in time it does begin to thicken meaningfully, go ahead and pour the nearly saponified batch, and allow the soap a normal cure period. Hope for the best, but be prepared for unusable soap. Some super-fatted vegetable soap formulas, made with high percentages of unsaturated oils, with

Trouble Sign	Reasons Why	What to Do
Mixture in pan not tracing (continued)		no more than 20 percent coconut oil, with a minimum requirement of sodium hydroxide, and without palm oil or tallow, can be made over a ten to sixteen hour period, using a casual stir method. But the recipes in this book are formulated to saponify within seven to forty minutes; hours and hours of processing would signal a problem.
Curdled mixture (small, pearly pebbles forming near the bottom of the pan)	◆ Oils, lye, or both poured at too high a temperature ◆ Irregular stirring ◆ Stirring process was too slow	Pour the soap mixture once it has saponified, but if the final soaps are filled with these irregularities (and they probably will be), do not use the final bars.
Slightly grainy mixture	◆ Soap was made using temperatures which were very high or very low ◆ Stirring process was not brisk and constant	This is an aesthetic problem only.
Mixture in pan beginning to set up prematurely (seizing)	◆ Temperatures used were too high or too low ◆ Fats/oils are overreacting to synthetic fragrance ◆ Fats/oils are overreacting to certain pure essential oils, like clove or cassia ◆ High percentage of pomace olive oil or tallow in formula	Carefully, but quickly, pour soap mixture into the frames, using a spatula to scoop out the firmer soap. Do your best to level the soap in the frame, as you would spread cake batter toward the edges of a cakepan. Proceed as usual.
Mixture in pan suddenly begins to streak	◆ Synthetic fragrance oils made with alcohol or dipropylene glycol were used to scent the soap ◆ Soapmaking temperatures were too cold	If the mixture seems otherwise correct, and it has saponified, quickly pour the soap mixture into the frame. This is an aesthetic problem only, with what you might even consider to be an interesting design within the final bars.

DIAGNOSING SIGNS OF TROUBLE IN THE FINAL SOAPS

Trouble Sign	Reasons Why	What to Do
Soaps marbled with white streaks (a swirled design; not solid white pieces)	◆ Uneven emulsion from uneven stirring ◆ Temperatures of oils and lye too cold ◆ Synthetic fragrance oils used to scent the soap ◆ Stirred too long after adding fragrance	Be sure that these white swirls are not shiny, alkaline chunks of lye. Swirls created by the fragrance do not effect the purity of the soap.
Soft, spongy soap	◆ Not enough sodium hydroxide	You can try to cure these for a longer period (a few more weeks), but it is unlikely that these will become firm enough for bar soap.
Hard, brittle soap	◆ Too much sodium hydroxide	Do not use these bars. They are probably quite alkaline, with a significant excess of sodium hydroxide.
Cosmetic air bubbles	◆ Stirred too long (soap should have been poured into the frames sooner) ◆ Stirred too quickly, more like whipping or beating	Be sure that these holes are not filled with lye. If they are just air bubbles, the soaps are fine.
Separation — greasy layer (unsaponified oils) on top of hard soap (harsh soap with excess lye)	◆ Insufficient stirring ◆ Inaccurate proportion of fats/oils to sodium hydroxide (too much sodium hydroxide) ◆ Too quick a temperature drop in the frames ◆ Soap poured into frames too soon	Do not use these. Parts of these bars will be highly alkaline. Consider these unsafe for personal use.
Hard soap with bright white areas (not streaks, but random chunks of slippery solid lye)	◆ Too much sodium hydroxide used ◆ Stirring process was too slow or inconsistent	Do not use these bars — the chunks of lye will burn.
Excessive amount of white powder on top of bars, or cakey, crumbly slab of soap	◆ Too much sodium hydroxide ◆ Hard water used to dissolve the sodium hydroxide	Do not use these bars. They are highly caustic.

DIAGNOSING SIGNS OF TROUBLE IN THE FINAL SOAPS

Trouble Sign	Reasons Why	What to Do
Mottled soap with an irregular freckled look	◆ Uneven stirring ◆ Fats or oils exposed to radical temperature changes during refinement or packaging	Proceed with process. This is an aesthetic problem only.
While cutting the few-days-old soap into bars, the knife meets with resistance in certain spots. Upon careful inspection, soaps have hard, shiny, white chunks of solid lye surrounding areas of normal soft soap and are wet underneath with a slippery liquid lye that soaks through the waxed-paper onto the soap frames.	◆ Poured soap into frames before saponification was complete ◆ Stirring process too slow and inconsistent	Do not use these bars — they are caustic.
Cracks in soaps	◆ Too much sodium hydroxide ◆ Too much stirring, more like beating or whipping ◆ Soap set too quickly	If these seem harsh, too much sodium hydroxide makes these unusable. If the cracks are temperature related, the problem is only an aesthetic one.
Soap takes over three days to harden considerably (following the covered insulation period)	◆ Not enough sodium hydroxide ◆ Citrus oils slowing down the process slightly ◆ Curing soap exposed to extreme temperatures and/or drafts ◆ High percentage of castor oil with an insufficient amount of sodium hydroxide	Allow the bars a few more weeks to cure. Do not use them if they never firm up sufficiently.

DIAGNOSING SIGNS OF TROUBLE IN THE FINAL SOAPS

Trouble Sign	Reasons Why	What to Do
Lye pockets (air bubbles filled with liquid or powdered lye)	◆ Insufficient stirring ◆ Too much sodium hydroxide ◆ Stirring process too slow	These bars are unsafe — the pockets of lye will burn.

IF IN DOUBT, TEST FOR PH

If you are at all uncertain of your diagnostic ability, purchase a pH test kit and test the soaps yourself. Wait until the bars have cured, about three to six weeks after they were cut and trimmed. If you are concerned about particular areas on the bars, test these directly.

Aubrey Hampton, in his book *Natural Organic Hair and Skin Care,* discusses pH and stresses that a wide range of values can be acceptable for skin-care products. He wrote that the skin can adjust to a pH of 8.0–10.5 more easily than it can to the synthetic chemicals which are added to lower pH. The term "pH balanced," like so many advertising gimmicks, has been exploited; a neutral (7.0) reading does not reveal enough about a product.

A range of 5.5–10.5 seems to be an acceptable range for hair and skin products; be aware that pH readings may vary somewhat from test to test. I aim for a range of 5.5 to 8.0. Aim for a range rather than a precise number. If you have any doubt about a soap, do not use it.

Though pH tests serve a purpose, they do have their limitations. I have noticed that even when a bar of soap tests within the neutral range, the soap solution (some soap dissolved in water) can test slightly alkaline. Do monitor the bars, but aim for a safe range, not just one specific value.

CAUTION
Never pour raw soap down the drain.

CHAPTER 11
Cutting and Trimming

There are several different methods you can use to slice a block of soap into bars, depending upon the type of mold used and the variety of soap. Some soapmakers like to pour into a towerlike rectangular mass, and then use a cheesewire to slice this block into layers and bars. Others, like myself, prefer to pour the soap into a one layer thick rectangle. Once the soap is firm enough, this mass needs only to be sliced lengthwise and crosswise, brownie-style. In my opinion, this method allows the soapmaker more control and precision, as it requires less dexterity than the three-dimensional tower. I figure that the fewer cuts I have to make, the greater the odds of my winding up with fairly even bars of soap. I have more control over a knife than I do a piece of cheesewire or fishing line.

WHEN TO CUT

Though each batch of soap is unique, most of the recipes in this book will produce soap which will harden enough to slice within one to seven days. Once moderately firm pressure (using your fingertip) meets with resistance, your soap is ready to be sliced. For a vegetable soap made with a high percentage of coconut and palm oils, this is usually soon after the twenty-four-hour insulation period, or within a few days.

Deep inside, the soap will still be somewhat soft, but the bars will harden fully as more surfaces are exposed. Soaps or shampoo bars which incorporate a large quantity of citrus oils can take longer to harden. Also, formulas which include a high percentage of unsaturated oils can take a few extra days.

HOW TO CUT

First, I slice the bars lengthwise and crosswise. Mark each side of the tray with permanent marker at the correct measure, every three inches on the ends and every 2⅜ inches on the sides. Then lay a ruler on top of the soap, and connect the opposite sides by cutting a slight impression along the length of the ruler using a paring knife. Once all of these lighter cuts are made, check for precision, and then use the paring knife to completely cut all the way through the soap along the lines drawn.

CURING THE BARS

After the soap is cut into bars, lift the entire mass out of the tray, holding on to the waxed paper for leverage. Pull the waxed paper away from the sides of bars and flatten it against the work surface. Gently peel each bar off the paper, taking care not to press too hard — remember that the bars are not completely firm. Using the paring knife, slice about ¹⁄₁₆ inch off the top of each bar to remove the thin layer of soda ash which forms on the surface of the soap mass. This is one of my favorite steps, for as this dull, matted finish is sliced away, the rich, uniform piece of soap below is finally unveiled.

The soaps are not yet finished, however. Stacking the soaps to complete their cure-time is as important as all of the other parts of the process. The bars still are slightly alkaline at this point and they must be handled carefully to avoid discoloration and rancidity. I do not stack the soaps, brick-style, as other manuals have suggested, for they ideally need complete exposure, with no contact with other bars.

Sometimes I lay the bars on wicker or rattan placemats. Plain brown paper grocery bags are wonderful for single layer drying. Do not use the printed side, as the alkaline bars will pick up the dye. Each bag will hold 20 four-ounce bars, and the dry, porous paper allows even the bottoms of the bars to breathe. Set these bags in a somewhat cool, dust-free environment on a shelf or a table. (Closets and drawers do not allow for enough circulation for maximum protection against rancidity.) Wait three to four weeks before wrapping the bars.

DECORATIVE MOLDING

This book is about bar soaps, but I encourage you to make soap balls occasionally for fun — especially if you've got children who want to try their hand at soapmaking. After about a week of curing inside of the frame, the soap should be firm enough to shape by hand. If not, wait a few days longer. Without painstaking attention to symmetry, slice the batch into 40 bars, slice off the thin layer of soda ash, then, wearing flexible gloves, hand-form each bar into a large soapball. Cure for the remaining few weeks, as described above for bar soaps.

All-vegetable soap does not lend itself particularly well to decorative molding. Though it eventually hardens nicely, it is not rock hard within a day, as the best soaps for molding are. Tallow/vegetable combinations harden quickly and release from the mold with all of their edges and fine detail intact. An all-palm oil soap, or even a soap made with other vegetable oils, but primarily of palm and coconut oils, could be molded. But the skin-care quality of the soap would be inferior to a carefully designed blend.

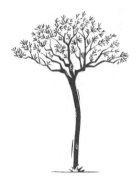

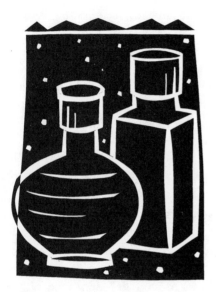

Beyond

The

Basics

PART

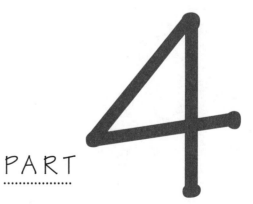

CHAPTER 12
Creative Ideas for Wrapping Soap

$\mathcal{S}$ometimes I almost hate to wrap my soaps, because I've noticed that the prettier the wrapping, the less likely people are to unwrap and use the bars. I've been told that many of my bars sit on bathroom counters and shelves for months because "they're just too pretty to open." One friend no longer even notices that the bars I gave her a year ago still sit on her living room coffee table, directly in front of us as we chat.

As you consider the following options, be thinking about the odds and ends you have around the house which can be recycled to wrap soap. Some of the seemingly outrageous ideas often turn out to be favorites.

WRAPPING SUGGESTIONS

Fold lightweight fabric squares like wrapping paper around the bar. Holding the bottom ends in place, tie four or five strands of raffia in one bundle lengthwise across the bar, in a shoelace bow. Tie another four or five strands crosswise in the same manner, using a tight knot to keep the loops in place. Fluff out the strands and loops casually and attach dried flowers, like statice, gomphrena, or rosebuds, with a hot glue gun to the center of the bar (figure 1, A–C).

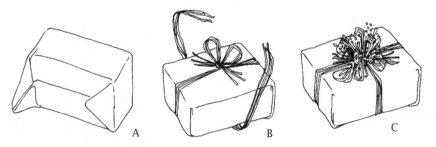

Figure 1.

Center a strip of simple or decorative paper on the bar, wrap the strip around the bar, and glue the edges together, leaving both ends of the soap exposed. Use either a professionally

136

printed label or your own hand-drawn design. You might design an image that reflects something special about your soap (figure 2).

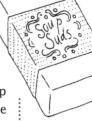

Figure 2.

Stamp a plain square of white muslin using a favorite stamp and fabric ink, then center the soap in the middle of the unprinted side and fold package-style. Be sure that the stamp is situated nicely on the top of the bar before glueing the bottom edges to one another with fabric glue (figure 2).

Sew a drawstring fabric pouch using a 4-inch by 10-inch piece of tightly woven lace, or another fabric for the pouch. Cut a 10- to 12-inch length of lace seam binding or a strip of finish-

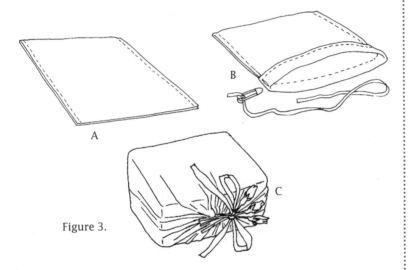

Figure 3.

ing lace for the drawstring. Fold the wide piece of lace in half, right sides together. Stitch up the sides. Fold the top edge inward, leaving a 1- inch seam. Stitch a ¾- inch seam to hold the drawstring, leaving a ½- inch opening. Using a safety pin, ease the seam binding into the seam allowance, and tie the lace into a bow or a loop. Turn inside out and tuck soap into the pouch. Attach some dried rosebuds, or other dried flowers, for a final touch (figure 3, A–C).

Find a favorite sponge (huge natural elephant ear sponges and loofah work nicely) and carefully slice into the sponge with

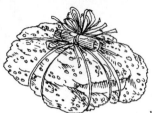

Figure 4.

an exacto knife, or sharp scissors, removing a piece from the middle. Tuck your soap into the slit and wrap the sponge with natural raffia. For a special addition, tuck a small bottle of herbal almond oil into the raffia loops and secure well (figure 4).

Set a bar of soap in a small wicker soapdish or basket and wrap with cellophane, or leave the bar exposed, wrapping only with raffia and dried herbs, flowers, or baby pine cones (figure 5).

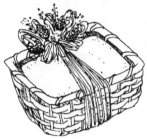

Figure 5.

Wrap soap in a natural cloth, like hempcloth, and tie with raffia, ribbon, or braided cord. Tuck in some dried flowers or herbs (figure 6).

Tuck a bar of soap into a pretty soap mitt, fold the open end over, and secure with a carefully disguised safety pin. Attach a small gift tag, preferably hand drawn.

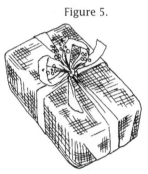

Figure 6.

Make a unique baby gift by tucking extra mild soaps into a pretty basket, along with a few creatively folded hunks of natural cloth, like hempcloth. Weave raffia, cord, or ribbons through the basket material, and tuck in a drawing of a nature scene printed on recycled paper. Decorate with gentle, natural colors, skipping the candy pinks and blues (figure 7).

Serve your soap as brownie bars by spreading a pretty linen dish towel onto a decorative platter, then lay a variety of soap bars, brownie-style, on top of the cloth. Cover the bars with the corners of the cloth (four triangles folded over inward). Attach a card to the cloth, warning that these bars are to be served in the bath and the shower.

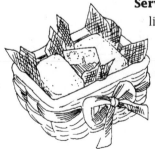

Figure 7.

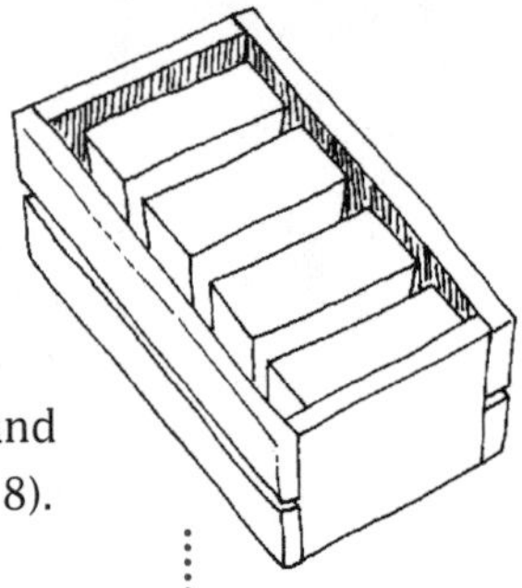

Fill wooden crates with a variety of soap bars,
either wrapped or unwrapped. Alternating the natural color variations makes a beautiful arrangement.
Weave raffia in and out of the wooden slats of the crate and
attach some dried botanicals with a hot glue gun (figure 8).

Figure 8.

Make dinner party favors by wrapping soaps with fabrics, or
even beautiful paper dinner napkins. Dainty fabric ribbons or
bows can be glued gently to the napkins, or wrap with splashy
foil strands.

Use plain brown parcel paper folded around the soap like a
package and tied with the natural color raffia or rough twine.
Use a hot glue gun to attach small pine cones and dried flowers
and herbs.

Make an accordion wrap by folding a large piece of solid-col-
ored, fine-quality paper, accordion style, then place the soap in
the center of the wrong side. Wrap as you would wrap a small
package, folding the sides over the bar first, and then fold and
tape or glue the ends in place. The narrower pleats keep all of
them in place. Also, by folding the paper tightly against the
bars, the pleats stay in place better. Use fabric glue to secure the
bottom edges together and decorate with dried botanicals using
a hot glue gun (figure 9, A–C).

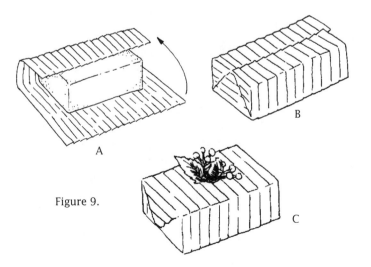

A

B

Figure 9.

C

Wrap soap in a paper doily, without large holes; then tie and bow lengthwise and crosswise with lace seam binding. Glue rosebuds or other dried flowers onto the doily.

Make use of some unusual gift wrapping paper to wrap the soap package-style, then tie with many strands (4 or 5 for each direction) of ribbon. Curl each individual ribbon strand with scissors. Decorate with bows, party favors or balloons, and tie a gift card to the ribbon strands through a punched hole in the card.

Use washi paper instead of fabric to wrap your soap. Washi is an expensive Japanese paper made from quality plant fibers. It is a porous flexible weave which wraps gently and easily around the soap, into a variety of folded styles. Wrap washi around the soap, using ideas from this chapter and from the book *Gift Wrapping: Creative Ideas from Japan* (see page 172). Tie some of these designs with *mizuhiki,* a multicolored Japanese cord, for a festive holiday look. (See page 161 for information on how to order washi and mizuhiki.)

Make a strand of soapballs by laying two rectangular sheets of washi or fabric on top of one another, wrong sides together. Trim the short ends with pinking shears (figure 10A). Keeping a 2-inch border at both ends, space the soap balls evenly across the lower longer edge (figure 10B). Wrap the bottom edge over the tops of the soap balls and continue rolling up the paper or fabric slowly (figure 10C). Tie the ends with string, then tie between the other soap balls. Finally, tie and bow pretty ribbon, raffia, mizuhiki, lace, or braided cord over the string (figure 10D).

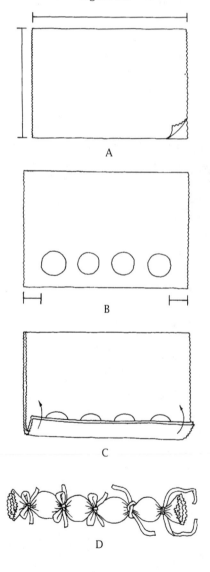

Figure 10.

A

B

C

D

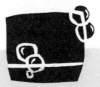

A Soapmaker's Story
Karen Voigts/Maple Hill Farm

In the early 1980s, Karen and Tom Voigts moved from the city to a small farm in Michigan with a deserted barn that looked ready to be revived. Karen and Tom had no experience in animal husbandry. Their son was allergic to cow's milk, so a goat became the animal of choice. "Goats seemed like such friendly animals, and we could see how well our son could tolerate goat milk," recounts Karen. "We settled on raising a goat, but soon discovered that goats are too sociable to be alone, so we had to get another."

By spring, with newborn kid goats, Karen and Tom had more goat milk than they could possibly use. Karen tried to use it up, making ice cream, custards, cheeses, and fudge. Then, one day, she saw a recipe for goat-milk soap in a magazine. "Wow!" she says. "Another way to use goat milk!"

"Aunt Karen's Goat Milk Soap" is made with lard, tallow, coconut and olive oils, and pure essential oils. Karen also makes "Goat Milk Shaving Soap," sold as a refill, or as part of a shaving-soap set, with mug, brush, and round soap. Karen searched long and hard to find suppliers who offer preservative-free fats and oils. She uses no artificial coloring; instead, when she wants to color her holiday bars, she adds liquid chlorophyll for a festive, green soap.

Their soap is made in Karen and Tom's big country kitchen, with pure, fresh goat milk. Though their soapmaking business has grown from local sales to nationwide distribution through wholesaling and retail mail order, "we still manufacture our soap in the same handcrafted manner, because we find that people are always searching for handmade quality products," says Karen.

Three Furoshiki Wrappings

A furoshiki is a piece of fabric wrapped to form a carrying handle within the design. This works well for wrapping a single soapball in washi or fabric.

Method 1 (for a single soap ball)

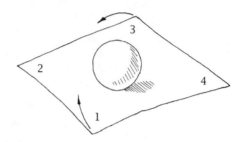

1. Lay the fabric square with one corner directly in front of you. Lay the soap ball in the middle of the fabric.

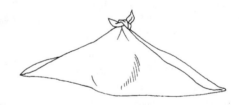

2. Tie the tips of corners 1 and 3 in a knot, with just ½-inch of material hanging from the knot to make knot 1–3.

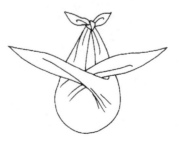

3. Then cross corner 2 over corner 4, over the front top of the soapball.

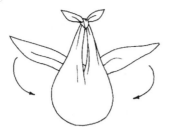

4. Turn the ball around and bring the loose ends around to tie snugly against the top surface of the soapball, enclosing the lower part of knot 1–3.

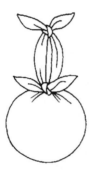

5. Pull knot 1–3 up through knot 2–4, tightening the material around the soapball to form a little carrying handle .

Method 2 (for a single soap ball)

1. Lay the fabric square with one corner pointing directly toward you. Place the soap ball in the middle of the fabric.

2. Tie the tips of corners 1 and 2 in a knot, allowing just ½ inch of material hanging from the knot.

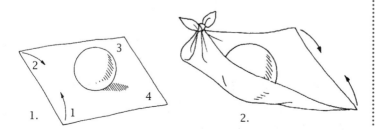

3. Tie corners 3 and 4 in the same way. Pull knot 1–2 under knot 3–4, making the fabric fit snugly around the soap ball.

4. The fabric should thoroughly cover the soap ball, with the knotted loop forming a carrying handle on top.

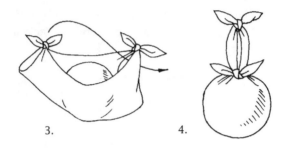

3. 4.

Method 3 (for a bar of soap)
Make a scarf wrap using linen, silk, washi, or any free-flowing fabric with finished edges (kerchiefs, bandannas, or scarves work nicely).

1. Lay the fabric square with one corner pointing toward you. Lay the soap in the front third of the fabric, with one of the shorter edges of the rectangle facing you.

2. Bring corner 1 up over the soap to just reach the other top edge of the soap.

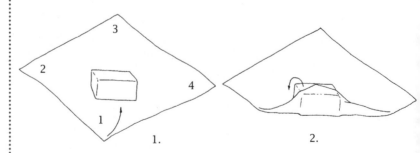

1. 2.

3. Holding the fabric in place, roll the bar over, along with the fabric, one or two times toward the opposite corner of the fabric (corner 3), until just a bar and a half of fabric length remains.

4. Fold corner 3 toward you, over the side of the bar nearest you.

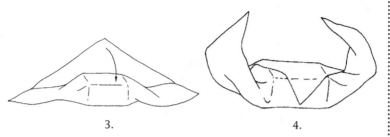

3.　　　　　　　　　　4.

5. Lift corners 2 and 4 and tie a knot, crossing corner 2 over and under corner 4.

6. Complete the knot by moving corner 2 back over and under corner 4 and pulling both ends to tighten the knot.

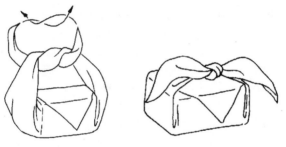

5.　　　　　　　　　　6.

A Soapmaker's Story
Sandy Maine/SunFeather Herbal Soap Company

In 1979, Sandy Maine was working as an Adirondack Wilderness guide when she decided that a second occupation was needed to round out her irregular schedule. It was then that the idea for SunFeather Herbal Soap Company came to her one morning. "Off I went to my dear grandmother, whose stories of making soap had always intrigued me," says Sandy. Grandma and I made it a day of soap research — from Olga Nielsen's kitchen, over to Helen Sorenson's, and then to Mrs. Jorgensen's basement, where a forty-year-old bar of `Granny Soap' was unearthed."

Sandy spent the following six months in search of the perfect soap recipe. "Libraries, bookstores, antique book shops from Peabody's in Baltimore to the Smithsonian, ... no stone was left unturned." Then she stumbled upon Ann Bramson's book, *Soap: Making It, Enjoying It,* and read it cover to cover without interruption. That night, Sandy made her twentieth test batch of soap. "The following day, I turned a perfect chunk of soap out onto the counter of my farmhouse kitchen with a great thump." says Sandy.

The next five years were spent building a company. As SunFeather grew more labor intensive, Sandy's wheels were spinning, thinking of labor-saving equipment. Sandy, and her resourceful husband and friends, designed collapsible molds, large drying racks, hydraulic hand-operated cutting machines, and pot-tipping girdles. When Sandy started out in 1979, she knew of no other soapmakers. Resources were scarce — building SunFeather was truly a pioneer effort.

Today, SunFeather operates out of approximately 5,000 square feet in a renovated bar. "SunFeather has evolved from a one-person operation to a family of sixteen women, all performing different, yet complementary, roles," says Sandy. "The women who work at `The Soap Shop' describe work as having a family feeling."

SunFeather's products reflect Sandy's philosophy, which she has always shared with other start-up soapers. "I have always tried to encourage people to `go for it,' but please do it your own way!" SunFeather's unique approach includes donating a portion of each sale of selected bars to assist different environmental and peace organizations.

SunFeather makes 100-pound batches of soap from olive, coconut, palm and castor oils, and both essential and fragrance oils. The natural color sources include clays, seaweeds, dried botanicals, grains, fruits, and root and spice powders.

They also sell soapmaking kits for beginners and distribute raw materials (fats, oils, essential and fragrance oils, sodium hydroxide, french clay powder, comfrey root powder), and supplies (thermometers, soapmaking books, and molds). Sandy urges all soapmakers to use well-calibrated scales and thermometers and to pay exact attention to detail.

Sandy has enjoyed watching this grassroots industry take hold and she encourages all new soapmakers to be creative and autonomous, rather than simply reproduce someone else's creations. "Thankfully, soap is a consumable product, and there's *lots* of market to share!" exclaims Sandy. She is finishing up a book entitled *The Soap Book* and is also designing a soapmaking video. Both works are sure to educate and inspire.

CHAPTER 13
The Chemistry of Soapmaking

Chemistry can be intimidating. However, it is possible for a layperson to learn enough about chemistry to become a better soapmaker without becoming an expert, and without becoming bored!

After reading this chapter, you should:

◆ Have a good feel for the basic chemical equation in soapmaking.

◆ Understand how to use certain scientific charts to predict the soap characteristics produced by various fats and oils.

◆ Understand how to use the SAP Value Chart to determine the approximate amount of sodium hydroxide you will need for a particular soap formula. You do not have to understand the chemistry to make soap, but the knowledge is helpful and can even be fun.

THE BASIC CHEMICAL REACTION

The soapmaking process is simply the combination of an acid and a base to form a salt. Something acidic combines with something alkaline to form something neutral — in this case, a mild bar of soap. In soapmaking, the oils and fats are the acids, sodium hydroxide is the base also known as the alkali, and soap is the salt of the particular acids used.

Consider, first, the chemical makeup of the fats and oils. For the cold-process soapmaker, each fat or oil consists of a different combination of triglycerides, compounds made up of three so-called *fatty acids,* linked to one molecule of glycerol (a form of glycerin). For example, *olein* is a triglyceride consisting of three molecules of oleic acid and one molecule of glycerol. A fatty acid is a different combination of carbon, hydrogen, and oxygen atoms. For example, oleic acid is a fatty acid consisting of 18 carbon atoms, 34 hydrogen atoms, and 2 oxygen atoms. Most often, a triglyceride contains two or three different fatty acids, rather than three of the same kind.

Consider, next, the chemical makeup of the base. For the cold-process soapmaker, the common base is sodium hydroxide. Sodium hydroxide is a combination of one sodium ion and one hydroxide ion. The hydroxide ion consists of one oxygen atom and one hydrogen atom. It is the hydroxide ion, not the sodium ion, which is most critical to soapmaking. Other bases could be used instead of sodium hydroxide, because, again, it is the hydroxide ion which reacts with the acid to make soap.

Stirring the mixture is critical, and directly affects the time required for saponification. Though it is possible to have a few momentary breaks in stirring, consistent, brisk stirring allows the free fatty acids to continue to react with the free alkali. Without this nearly constant contact of the reactive ingredients, the process slows down.

When fats and oils react with sodium hydroxide, what is really happening is that triglycerides are releasing glycerin, permitting the remaining fatty acids (so-called *free fatty acids)* to combine with hydroxide ions to form soap.

Note that in cold-process soapmaking, the glycerol attached to the fatty acid is released and remains in the soap in the form of glycerin. Glycerin is a marvelous additive which moisturizes the skin. Industrial manufacturers either remove this glycerin and sell it as a by-product, or make soap with free fatty acids (without glycerin) rather than with triglycerides (which include glycerin). This is just one more reason why homemade soap can be so much finer.

USING SCIENTIFIC CHARTS TO MIX FATS AND OILS

The major characteristics we look for in a soap — the hardness of the bar, the fluffiness of the lather, and the stability of the lather — depend upon which fatty acids are involved. Each fat or oil is a unique combination of several different fatty acids. The characteristics contributed by a particular fat or oil are determined by the characteristics of its predominant fatty acid(s). For example, palm oil consists of 40.1 percent palmitic acid — a fatty acid which increases the hardness of a bar. That's why palm oil is known for contributing to a hard soap. Once you know the fatty acid makeup of the fats or oils in a soap formula, you can figure out what characteristics the soap will have. The following charts will assist you in this process.

As these charts indicate, no one fat or oil has all of the

characteristics soapmakers find desirable in their soap. Thus, soapmakers must combine different fats and oils to produce the desired outcome. This is where the skill and artistry of the soapmaker is most tested. Mixing fats and oils also affects the amount of sodium hydroxide required to properly complete the reaction, as discussed on page 155.

USING THE SAP VALUE CHART

THE FATTY-ACID MAKEUP OF SOME COMMON FATS AND OILS

FAT OR OIL	FATTY ACID (IN PERCENTAGES)
Babassu Oil	Lauric 44.1/Oleic 16.1/Myristic 15.4/Palmitic 8.5/Capric 6.6/Capryli 4.8/Stearic 2.7/Linoleic 1.4/Arachidic .2/Caproic .2
Castor Oil	Ricinoleic 87/Oleic 7.4/Linoleic 3.1/Lauric Myristic Palmitic and Stearic 2.4
Coconut Oil	Lauric 45.4/Myristic 18.0/Palmitic 10.5/Capric 8.4/Oleic 7.5/Capryli 5.4/Stearic 2.3/Caproic .8/Arachidic .4/ Palmitoleic .4/Linoleic (trace)
Olive Oil	Oleic 84.4/Palmitic 6.9//Linoleic 4.6/Stearic 2.3/Arachidic .1/Myristic (trace)
Palm Oil	Oleic 42.7/Palmitic 40.1/Linoleic 10.3/Stearic 5.5/Myristic 1.4
Soybean Oil	Linoleic 50.7/Oleic 28.9/Palmitic 9.8/Linolenic 6.5/Stearic 2.4/Arachidic .9/Palmitoleic .4/Lauric .2/Myristic .1/C_{14} monoethenoic .1
Beef Tallow	Oleic 49.6/Palmitic 27.4/Stearic 14.1/Myristic 6.3/Linoleic 2.5

SOAP CHARACTERISTICS PRODUCED BY VARIOUS FATTY ACIDS

Fatty Acid	Hard Bar	Cleansing	Fluffy Lather	Conditioning	Stable Lather
Lauric	X	X	X		
Palmitic	X				X
Stearic	X				X
Ricinoleic			X	X	X
Oleic		X		X	
Linoleic		X		X	

MOLECULAR WEIGHTS OF FATTY ACIDS

If you know the molecular weight of a fatty acid in your soap, often you can predict the lathering ability of your soap. In general, the greater the molecular weight of a fatty acid, the less fluffy and more stable the lather.

For example, beef tallow makes a thin lather. It consists of 24.6 percent of palmitic acid and 30.5 percent of stearic acid which have relatively high molecular weights of 256 and 284.

The molecular weight chart can help predict other soap characteristics as well. In general, as molecular weight increases, a fatty acid's cleansing capability decreases, its potential to cause skin irritation decreases, and its hardness increases. Also, and the significance of this will be discussed below, the greater the molecular weight, the lower the SAP value.

Fatty Acid	Formula	Molecular Weight
Butyric	$C_4H_8O_2$	88
Capric	$C_{10}H_{20}O_2$	172
Caproic	$C_6H_{12}O_2$	116
Lauric	$C_{12}H_{24}O_2$	200
Linoleic	$C_{18}H_{32}O_2$	280
Myristic	$C_{14}H_{28}O_2$	228
Oleic	$C_{18}H_{34}O_2$	282
Palmitic	$C_{16}H_{32}O_2$	256
Ricinoleic	$C_{18}H_{34}O_3$	298
Stearic	$C_{18}H_{36}O_2$	284

IODINE VALUE OF FATS AND OILS

The iodine value measures an oil's or fat's saturation. More specifically, it indicates the amount of iodine chloride the fat or oil could dissolve, expressed in centigrams of iodine dissolvable per gram of oil or fat. Saturated fats have low iodine values and unsaturated oils have high iodine values. Though exceptions occur, fats with low iodine values make the hardest soaps. Thus, for example, palm oil makes a hard soap and olive oil makes a softer soap.

Fat or Oil	Iodine Value (amount dissolved in centigrams/gram of oil)
Beef tallow	49.5
Lard oil	58.6
Babassu oil	15.5
Castor oil	85.5
Coconut oil	10.4
Olive oil	81.1
Palm oil	54.2
Palm kernel oil	37.0
Soybean oil	130
Peanut oil	93.4
Wheatgerm oil	125
Jojoba oil	85
Sweet almond oil	105
Kukui nut oil	165
Apricot kernel oil	102.5
Avocado oil	80

TO CALCULATE SODIUM HYDROXIDE

Each fat or oil has a saponification value (referred to as "SAP value"). The SAP value is actually a range of numbers, but the average of these numbers is usually presented on a chart. The SAP value of an oil or fat measures the amount of potassium hydroxide (chemical symbol KOH) in milligrams required to saponify (to react with and make soap out of) one gram of that oil or fat. So the SAP value divided by 1,000, multiplied by the weight of the oil equals the weight of potassium hydroxide required for saponification. For example, the SAP value of olive oil is 189.7. This means that 189.7 milligrams of KOH are required to completely saponify one gram (1,000 milligrams) of olive oil. The higher the SAP value, the more base required for saponification.

SAP VALUE CHART FOR COMMON FATS AND OILS

Fat or Oil	SAP Value
Beef tallow	197
Lard oil	194.6
Babassu oil	247
Castor oil*	180.3
Coconut oil	268
Olive oil	189.7
Palm oil	199.1
Palm kernel oil	219.9
Peanut oil	192.1
Soybean oil	190.6
Wheatgerm oil	185
Jojoba oil	97.5
Sweet almond oil	192.5
Kukui nut oil	190
Avocado oil	187.5
Apricot kernel oil	190
Shea butter (African karite butter)	180

Because of its higher molecular weight, castor oil has a lower SAP value and, in theory, requires less sodium hydroxide for saponification. But castor oil, with its high ricinoleic acid content, has its own set of rules. Ricinoleic acid has an unusual molecular arrangement, pulling castor oil into some additional bonding within the soap pan. More sodium hydroxide is required to accommodate the extra workload. When a formula calls for over 15 percent castor oil, use a discount of 5 percent, instead of a 15.5 percent discount (see box on page 154).

From the SAP value you can determine also how much sodium hydroxide (NaOH) is required for saponification, with some simple arithmetic and an understanding of basic soapmaking chemistry. Saponification is affected by the number of hydroxide ions in the solution. One molecule of sodium hydroxide (NaOH) has the same number of hydroxide ions (one) as one molecule of potassium hydroxide (KOH), but since KOH is heavier than NaOH, saponification requires less (by weight) of NaOH. More precisely, because the molecular weight of NaOH is 40 and the molecular weight of KOH is 56.1, the required weight of NaOH is $^{40}/_{56.1}$ of the required weight of KOH.

Weight of NaOH required = $^{40}/_{56.1}$ x weight of KOH required

Adjusting Calculations to Produce a Superfatted Soap

So far, the science and mathematics are reassuringly precise. Unfortunately, there is one additional complication which introduces some uncertainty. The above formula indicates how much sodium hydroxide is required to completely saponify an oil. However, the soapmaker does not want to completely saponify the fats and oils — you want *some* fat and oil to remain unsaponified. This makes the soap milder, less caustic, and more soothing.

Our skin's mantle is slightly acidic, anywhere between 4.00 and 6.75 on the pH scale (with pH 7 being neutral). Though our skin can tolerate a wide range of pH values, including some of the alkaline values, too much sodium hydroxide can be harsh. By using less sodium hydroxide than the SAP values suggest, and an excess of oils and nutrients, the bars are left with unsaponified oil within — this soap

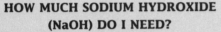

HOW MUCH SODIUM HYDROXIDE (NaOH) DO I NEED?

Suppose you want to saponify 10 pounds of olive oil. To figure how much sodium hydroxide is required, begin by looking up the SAP value.

Since the SAP value of olive oil is 189.7 (189.7 milligrams of KOH required per 1,000 milligrams of olive oil), multiply 10 pounds of olive oil by .1897; to figure the amount of potassium hydroxide (KOH) required — 1.897 pounds.

The next step is to multiply the amount of KOH required by the fraction $^{40}/_{56.1}$ to figure the amount of sodium hydroxide required — 1.35 pounds.

The final step is to multiply the amount of sodium hydroxide required for complete saponification by 84.5 percent (or whatever discount you find works), to produce a superfatted soap.

is gentle and moisturizing. See page 131 for more information on pH values.

The question is, how much less sodium hydroxide should be used? That is, after applying the formula on page 154 and determining a precise amount of sodium hydroxide for complete saponification, how much should the precise amount be discounted? I cannot give you a neat answer here. I have searched for a single discount I could apply consistently, but haven't come up with one. I've worked with discounts ranging from 7 percent to 20 percent. The bigger the discount, the less base used, resulting in a milder soap that will also become rancid more quickly. When I do my calculations for a new soap formula, I usually begin with a 15.5 percent discount. This will provide a good approximation of the amount of sodium hydroxide required, but you will still have to experiment.

Working with a Combination of Oils

The SAP value calculations outlined earlier were for saponifying a single oil. But a soapmaker will never use just a single fat or oil — you always will be combining fats and oils to achieve a desired effect. To determine how much base to use in a soap formula with several fats and oils, you must calculate the SAP value for the entire mixture of fats and oils. A simple weighted average calculation can be made, as follows.

Suppose a soapmaker wishes to combine five pounds of olive oil, three pounds of coconut oil, and two pounds of palm oil. How much sodium hydroxide should be used? The following are the steps to take to figure this amount:

1. Determine the SAP value for the mixture of oils. Using the SAP value chart and the percentage by weight each oil contributes to the whole mixture, calculate the combined SAP value.

$$.5(189.7) + .3(268) + .2(199.1) = 215$$

2. Multiply the total weight of the oils by the combined SAP value to determine the amount of potassium hydroxide required.

(10 pounds) by .215 (215 divided by 1000) = 2.15 pounds

3. Multiply 2.15 pounds (the pounds of potassium hydroxide required) by the fraction $^{40}\!/_{56.1}$ to determine the pounds of sodium hydroxide required for complete saponification.

2.15 pounds x $^{40}\!/_{56.1}$ = 1.53 pounds (of sodium hydroxide)

4. Multiply the result from Step 3 by 84.5 percent (to reflect the 15.5 percent reduction discount I typically apply to leave some unsaponified fats and oils) to find the final answer for the amount of sodium hydroxide required.

1.53 pounds x 84.5% = 1.29 pounds

Again, remember that this 15.5 percent reduction discount means that excess fat is left in the soap, too much of which causes rancidity. If you have this problem, you would notice it after six to twelve months. Fortunately, there's a solution. Adding preservatives — and natural preservatives are available — can postpone rancidity.

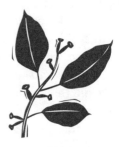

APPENDICES

A: SUPPLIERS

The following list continued to grow right up to the day of publication. To the best of my knowledge, there is no one, all-inclusive list of the manufacturers and distributors of the materials we're on the lookout for — including this one. Instead we must be detectives, always putting out feelers for a lower price, a better quality, and a reasonable minimum. Once in a while, another supplier will refer a competitor, or one of their customers. Occasionally, soapmakers will reveal their sources. And more often, the various trade journals will lead you to potential suppliers.

For us as cottage industry or home-soapmakers, the biggest problem is minimum orders. Most of the larger essential oil companies which offer the lower pricing require 5- to 30-pound minimums per essential oil. The huge distributors may even require the purchase of 55-gallon drums. The least expensive way to purchase palm oil is by tank truck, but how many of us can have 50,000 pounds pumped into the house? Palettes of drums (48 drums on a palette) are relatively inexpensive in comparison to gallons or pails of olive oil. The per pound cost for large quantities is dramatically cheaper than what most of us are used to paying for smaller quantities.

Ignorance can be bliss. Once I discovered how low it all can go, I've been a bit pained paying the higher prices, but I've shaved off some of the middleman costs by not going quite so far down the list of distributors. By the time we're purchasing from the fifth to the tenth customer of the original distributor, we're paying for many shipments and a whole lot of overhead. Each step closer to the manufacturer saves us something.

It's easier to start closer to the manufacturer and ask for customer referral than it is to start with the wholesale/retail distributors and ask for their suppliers. So don't be too discouraged if the huge companies won't do business with you. Explain your dilemma and ask for a list of customers in your area. The first couple of customer lists may be too large as well, but continue this process until you reach the right match for your personal needs.

Finally, watch for adulterated products. To increase profits, cheaper materials are added to the pure material, leaving the end user with an inferior product, one which will not react properly within the soap pan and one which degrades the quality we strive toward.

Ask questions, request a product analysis, pay for a chemical analysis, and take the time to call references to confirm quality and integrity. Something impure may still pass by us, but we increase our odds of success when we cover more bases and when we're alert.

Buyers' Guides

These two buyers' guides led me to many of the following suppliers. Smaller companies not listed in the directories are often customers of these larger companies. Ask the larger companies for some names of customers, if you cannot buy in the quantity they require.

International Buyers Guide
The Cosmetic, Toiletry, and Fragrance Association
1101 17th Street NW   Suite 300
Washington, DC 20036-4702
(202) 331-1770

DCI Directory Issue
Drug and Cosmetic Industry
Advanstar Communications, Inc.
1 East First Street
Duluth, Minnesota 55802
(218) 723-9477

Product Suppliers
Note: For company addresses and phone numbers, see pages 161–164.

Aloe Vera Gel
Desert Balm
Janca's Jojoba Oil and Seed Company
Lipo Chemicals, Inc.

Annatto Extract
(ask for pure oil-soluble)
Freeman Industries, Inc.
Penta Manufacturing Co.

Apricot Kernel Oil
Arista Industries, Inc.
Desert Balm
The Fanning Company
International Sourcing Inc.
Janca's Jojoba Oil and Seed Company
Jojoba Growers & Processors Inc.
Lebermuth Company
Liberty Natural Products, Inc.
Penta Manufacturing Company

Avocado Oil
Alban Muller International
Aphrodisia Products, Inc.
Arista Industries, Inc.
Croda Inc.
Desert Balm
The Fanning Company
Freeman Industries, Inc.
International Sourcing Inc.
Janca's Jojoba Oil & Seed Co.
Penta Manufacturing Co.
Welch, Holme & Clark Co., Inc.

Babassu Oil
Croda Inc.

Borage Oil
Croda Inc.
Desert Balm
Freeman Industries, Inc.

Borage Oil (continued)
International Sourcing Inc.
Janca's Jojoba Oil and Seed Company

Calendula Oil/Extract
(ask for pure oil-soluble)
Alban Muller International
Croda Inc.
Freeman Industries, Inc.

Carrot Root Oil/Carrot Seed Oil
International Sourcing Inc.
Janca's Jojoba Oil and Seed Company

Castor Oil
Alban Muller International
Arista Industries, Inc.
Frontier Cooperative Herbs
Janca's Jojoba Oil and Seed Company
Lebermuth Company
Liberty Natural Products, Inc.
Penta Manufacturing Co.

Chlorophyll
DeSouza's Food Corporation
Freeman Industries, Inc.
Penta Manufacturing Co.

Coconut Oil
Arista Industries, Inc.
Columbus Foods Company
The Fanning Co.
Janca's Jojoba Oil & Seed Co.
Liberty Natural Products Inc.
Penta Manufacturing Co.
Welch, Holme, and Clark Co., Inc.

Ecodermine
Sederma, Inc.

Essential Oils/Fragrance Oils
Aphrodisia Products Inc.
Belmay, Inc.

Creative Fragrances Manufacturing Inc.
Essential Oil Co.
The Fanning Company
Frontier Cooperative Herbs
Janca's Jojoba Oil and Seed Company
Lebermuth Company
Liberty Natural Products Inc.
Mountain Rose Herbs
Nectarine
Prima Fleur Botanicals Inc.
Robertet Inc.
Sweet Cakes Soaps & Sundries

Evening Primrose Oil
Arista Industries, Inc.
Croda Inc.
Desert Balm
Freeman Industries, Inc.
International Sourcing Inc.
Janca's Jojoba Oil and Seed Company

Grapefruit Seed Extract
Chemie Research & Manufacturing Co.,
    Inc.
Janca's Jojoba Oil and Seed Company
Liberty Natural Products Inc.

Jojoba Meal, Juniper Berry Meal, Flax Seed Meal
Janca's Jojoba Oil and Seed Company

Jojoba Oil
Arista Industries, Inc.
Desert Balm
Desert King Corporation
International Sourcing Inc.
Janca's Jojoba Oil & Seed Co.
Jojoba Growers & Processors, Inc.
Lebermuth Company
Lipo Chemicals, Inc.
Purcell Natural Jojoba (PNJ)

Kaolin

Aphrodisia Products Inc.
Janca's Jojoba Oil and Seed Company
Penta Manufacturing Co.
Whittaker, Clark & Daniels Inc.

Kukui Nut Oil

Alban Muller International
Arista Industries, Inc.
Desert Balm Essential Oil Co.
Freeman Industries, Inc.
The Hawaiian Kukui Nut Co.
International Sourcing Inc.
Janca's Jojoba Oil & Seed Co.

Lard

George A. Hormel & Co.
George Pfau's Sons & Co., Inc.
Stephenson Bros. & Co.

Montmorillonite/Bentonite

(known as French green clay)
Alban Muller
Southern Clay Products, Inc.

Olive Oil

Arista Industries, Inc.
Alban Muller International
Columbus Foods Company
Desert Balm Essential Oil Co.
The Fanning Company
Janca's Jojoba Oil and Seed Co.
Liberty Natural Products Inc.
Lipo Chemicals, Inc.
Penta Manufacturing Co.
Antonio Sofo & Son Importing
  Company
Welch, Holme & Clark Co., Inc.

Palm Kernel Oil

Penta Manufacturing Co.
Stevenson Brothers and Co.

Palm Oil

Alban Muller International
Arista Industries, Inc.
The Fanning Company
Liberty Natural Products Inc.
Penta Manufacturing Co.
Welch, Holme & Clark Co., Inc.

Peanut Oil

Arista Industries, Inc.
Desert Balm
The Fanning Company
Janca's Jojoba Oil & Seed Co.
Liberty Natural Products, Inc.
Penta Manufacturing Co.
Welch, Holme & Clark Co., Inc.

Plant Extracts

(ask for oil-soluble)
Alban Muller International
Freeman Industries, Inc.
Robertet Inc.

Rosa Mosqueta Rosehip Seed Oil

International Sourcing Inc.
Janca's Jojoba Oil and Seed Company

Seaweed (flakes, flour, and extracts)

International Sourcing Inc.

Shea Butter

Alban Muller International
Sederma, Inc.
Essential Oil Co.
International Sourcing Inc. (Ask them
  about their other exotic butters:
  Dhupa, Kokum, Mango, Mowrah, Sal,
  and Illipe)
Janca's Jojoba Oil & Seed Co.

Soapmaking Kits
Summers Past Farms
Sun Feather Herbal Soap Company

Soapmaking Molds
Essential Oil Company
Pourette Manufacturing Co.
The Soap Saloon

Sodium Hydroxide
American Research Products, Co.
Janca's Jojoba Oil and Seed Company
Penta Manufacturing Co.

Sweet Almond Oil
Alban Muller International
Aphrodisia Products Inc.
Arista Industries, Inc.
Desert Balm Essential Oil Co.
International Sourcing Inc.
Janca's Jojoba Oil & Seed Co.
Lebermuth Company
Liberty Natural Products, Inc.
Penta Manufacturing Co.
Welch, Holme & Clark Co., Inc.

Tallow
George Pfau's Sons Company, Inc.
Stephenson Brothers & Co.
Welch, Holme & Clark Co., Inc.

Tocopherols
Eastman Chemicals
Penta Manufacturing Co.

Vegetable Shortening
Alban Muller International
Arista Industries, Inc.
Desert Balm
Welch, Holme & Clark Co., Inc.

Washi and Mizuhiki
Kate's Paperie
Uwajimaya

Wheatgerm Oil
Arista Industries, Inc.
Desert Balm
The Fanning Company
Frontier Cooperative Herbs
Janca's Jojoba Oil and Seed Company
Liberty Natural Products, Inc.
Lipo Chemicals, Inc.
Penta Manufacturing Co.

Supplier Addresses

Alban Muller International
Distributed in the U.S. by TRI-K
Tri-K Industries
27 Bland Street
P.O. Box 312
Emerson, NJ 07630
(800) 526-0372
(201) 261-2800

**American Research Products
  Company**
30175 Solon Industrial Parkway
Solon, Ohio 44139
(800) 829-2802
(216) 349-1199

Aphrodisia Products Inc.
62 Kent Street
Brooklyn, NY 11222
(800) 221-6898
(718) 383-3677

Arista Industries, Inc.
1082 Post Road
Darien, CT 06820
(800) 637-6243
(203) 656-0328

Belmay, Inc.
200 Corporate Boulevard
South Yonkers, NY 10701
(914) 376-1515

Chemie Research & Manufacturing
160 Concord Drive
P.O. Box 181279
Casselberry, FL 32718-1279
(407) 831-4519

Columbus Foods Company Co., Inc.
800 N. Albany Avenue
Chicago, IL 60622
(800) 322-6457

Creative Fragrances Manufacturing Inc.
10890 Alder Circle
Dallas, TX 75238
(214) 341-3666

Croda, Inc.
7 Century Drive
Parsippany, NJ 07054
(201) 644-4900

Desert Balm
P.O. Box 4310
San Luis Obispo, CA 93403
(800) 729-2256

Desert King Corporation
3802 Main Street Suite 10
Chula Vista, CA 91911
(619) 427-7121

De Souza's Food Corporation
P.O. Box 395
Beaumont, CA 92223
(909) 849-5172

Eastman Chemical Co.
P.O. Box 431
Kingsport, TN 37662-5280
(800) EASTMAN
(615) 229-4006

Essential Oil Co.
P.O. Box 206
Lake Oswego, OR 97034
(800) 729-5912
(503) 697-5992

The Fanning Corporation
2450 W. Hubbard Street
Chicago IL 60612
(800) FANNING
(312) 248-5700

Freeman Industries, Inc.
100 Marbledale Road
Tuckahoe, NY 10707
(914) 961-2100
(800) 666-6454

Frontier Cooperative Herbs
3021 78th Street
P.O. Box 299
Norway, IO 52318
(800) 669-3275

George A. Hormel & Company
100 Corporate Drive
Lebanon, NJ 08833
(800) 320-4553
(908) 236-7009

Indiana Botanic Gardens Inc.
3140 E. Ridge Road
Hobrat, IN 46424
(219) 947-4040

International Sourcing Inc.
121 Pleasant Avenue
Upper Saddle River, NJ 07458
(800) 772-7672
(201) 934-8900

Janca's Jojoba Oil & Seed Co.
456 E. Juanita #7
Mesa, AZ 85204
(602) 497-9494

Jojoba Growers & Processors, Inc.
2267 South Coconino Drive
Apache Junction, AZ 85220
(602) 982-1125

Kate's Paperie
8 West 13th Street
New York, NY 10011
(212) 633-0570

Lebermuth Company
P.O. Box 4103
South Bend, IN 46634
(800) 648-1123
(219) 259-7000

Liberty Natural Products Inc.
8120 SE Stark
Portland, OR 97215
(800) 289-8427
(503) 256-1227

Lipo Chemicals, Inc.
207 19th Avenue
Paterson, NJ 07504
(201) 345-8600
(800) 347-LIPO

Mountain Rose Herbs
P. O. Box 2000
Redway, CA 95560
(800) 879-3337

Nectarine
1200 Fifth Street
Berkeley, CA 94710
(510) 528-0162

Oils of Aloha
66935 Kaukonahua Road
P.O. Box 685
Waialua, HI 96791
(800) 367-6010

Penta Manufacturing Company
P.O. Box 1448
Fairfield, NJ 07007
(201) 740-2300

George Pfau's Sons Co., Inc.
800 Wall Street
Jeffersonville, IN 47130
(800) PFAUOIL
(812) 283-6697

Pourette Manufacturing Co.
P.O. Box 15220
Seattle, WA 98115
(206) 525-4488
(800) 888-WICK

Prima Fleur Botanicals Inc.
12,01-R Andersen Drive
San Rafael, CA 94901
(415) 455-0957

Purcell Natural Jojoba
142 Front Street
Box 659
Avila Beach, CA 93424
(800) 676-1501
(805) 595-7275

Robertet, Inc.
125 Bauer Drive
P.O. Box 660
Oakland, NJ 07436-3190
(201) 337-7100

Sederma, Inc.
7110 Fort Hamilton Pkwy.
Brooklyn, NY 11228
(718) 833-1046

The Soap Saloon
7309 Sage Oak Court
Citrus Heights, CA 95621
(916) 723-6859

Antonio Sofo & Son Importing Company
253 Waggoner Blvd.
Toledo, OH 43612
(800) 447-4211

Southern Clay Products
1212 Church Street
Gonzales, TX 78629
(210) 672-2891
(800) 324-2891

Stevenson Brothers & Company
P.O. Box 38349
1039 West Venango Street
Philadelphia, PA 19140
(215) 223-2600

Summers Past Farms
15602 Old Hwy. 80
Flinn Springs, CA 92021
(800) 390-9969

Sweet Cakes Soaps & Sundries
39 Brookdale Road
Bloomfield, NJ 07003
(201) 338-9830

Uwajimaya
P.O. Box 3003
6th South and South King
Seattle, Washington 98114
(206) 624-6248

Welch, Holme & Clark Co., Inc.
7 Avenue L
Newark, NJ 07105-3805
(201) 465-1200

Whittaker, Clark & Daniels, Inc.
1000 Coolidge Street South
Plainfield, NJ 07080
(800) 732-0562

For small quantities at retail prices contact:

Sun Feather Herbal Soap Co.
1551 Highway 72
Potsdam, NY 13676
(315) 265-3648
(800) 771-SOAP

B: SOAPMAKING BUSINESSES

Patricia Arvidson/Island Soap
RFD Box 62
Brooksville, Maine 04617
(207) 326-9479

Barbara K. Bobo/Woodspirits Ltd., Inc.
1920 Apple Road
St. Paris, Ohio 43072
(513) 663-4327

Susan Miller Cavitch/Soap Essentials, Inc.
11150 Glen Birnham Road
Eads, Tennessee 38028

Catherine Failor/Copra Soaps
8926 N. Lombard
Portland, Oregon 97203
(503) 240-7494
(800) 364-4186

Jane Hawley/Nature's Acres
E. 8984 Weinke Road
North Freedom, WI 53951
(608) 522-4492

Camille Le Doux/Camille Le Doux's Handmade Soaps & Toiletries, Ltd.
108 Sunny Lane
Lafayette, LA 70506
(318) 988-4601

Sandie Ledray and Mary McIsaac/Brookside Soap Company
P.O. Box 55638
Seattle, Washington 98155
(206) 742-2265

Sandy Maine/SunFeather Herbal Soap Company
1551 Highway 72
Potsdam, NY 13676
(315) 265-3648
(800) 771-SOAP

Karen Voigts/Maple Hill Farm
1224 33rd Street Rt. 4
Allegan, MI 49010
(616) 673-6346

GLOSSARY
THE LANGUAGE OF SOAP

▼▼▼

Adulterate — To make impure by the addition of an inferior substance.

Alkali — A substance with a pH greater than 7. Sodium hydroxide is an example of an alkali (or a base) used to neutralize an acid to make soap.

Allergen — A substance which provokes an allergic reaction in the susceptible person, but can have no negative effect on another person.

Antibacterial — If a substance is antibacterial, it fights bacteria effectively.

Antioxidant — Oxidation occurs within fats and oils, as unattached oxygen molecules wander around and latch onto other molecules, forming unstable compounds. An antioxidant is a substance that inhibits oxygen from reacting with other molecules to form unstable compounds. Within soapmaking, antioxidants inhibit rancidity and spoilage of the fats and oils.

Antiseptic — A substance which slows the growth of microorganisms on living tissue. The following pure essential oils offer some antiseptic properties: cassia, clove, rosemary, thyme, sandalwood, and peppermint.

Aromatherapy — The art of using pure essential oils from plants for their physical and emotional therapeutic effects.

Astringent — A substance made mostly with witch hazel (natural) or isopropyl alcohol (synthetic) to remove soap film and dead skin. Thought to

contract tissues and close pores. Stick with the witch hazel solutions and use sparingly to avoid a drying effect.

Bacteriostatic — A substance which inhibits the growth of bacteria, but does not destroy bacteria.

Base — The alkali used within soapmaking which reacts with the fats or oils to form soap. Sodium hydroxide is the base used most often by the cold-process soapmaker.

Carcinogenic — A substance that causes some form of cancer.

Castile soap — A soap named for the region in Spain where it was first made. Once a pure olive oil soap, castile soap is now generally regarded as an olive/tallow combination.

Chlorophyll — The green matter found in the chloroplasts of plants, chlorophyll contributes antiseptic and antifungal properties to soap. It is also used as a natural colorant (pale green).

Clay — Mixture of natural minerals used in face masks to draw out impurities and excess sebum.

Coal tar — A tar obtained through the distillation of bituminous coal, used to make dyes and drugs. Many soapmakers use these synthetic dyes to color soap, though studies link coal tar dyes to cancer in animals and allergic reactions in humans; try to avoid them.

Cold-Process — The most simple soapmaking method; fats and oils react with lye to make soap and release glycerin, using no external heat once the ingredients have been blended.

Colorant — Perhaps not a generally accepted word, but adopted through use to mean a substance used to dye soaps naturally or synthetically. Non-synthetic examples include chlorophyll, cinnamon, turmeric, wheat germ oil, and herbal decoctions.

Cure — The process that soap bars experience over four to eight weeks as the soapmaking reaction continues within the final bars, leaving the soaps progressively less alkaline and more mild. Saponification, the soapmaking reaction, does not end once the liquid soap is poured into frames. As soaps cure, they are incorporating any remaining sodium hydroxide — changing from harsh to mild soaps.

Decoction — An extract obtained by covering roots and bark (tough-skinned botanicals) with water, and boiling down the liquid to a potent concentration. This is often used medicinally. Soapmakers use decoctions to color their soaps safely. Expect quiet, pale earth tones instead of bright synthetic colors.

Emollient — A substance spread onto the skin to hold in moisture and keep water loss to a minimum. Vegetable glycerin and vegetable oils are natural emollients; mineral oil has always been praised an an inexpensive natural emollient, but there is concern with respect to its petroleum base, which is thought to actually dry the skin over time.

Emulsion — The mixture of two incompatible substances by a third component (the emulsifier) which helps hold all three together in a unit.

Soap is an emulsifier, as it holds the dirt and oil in suspension in water. Oil and water are incompatible and soap holds them together; soap pulls the dirt and oils away from the skin and holds it to the water until a rinse washes the whole unit away.

Essential fatty acid — The few fatty acids which stand out above the others as especially effective are called essential fatty acids. Linoleic, linolenic, and arachidonic acids (known also as vitamin F) are essential fatty acids, those unsaturated fatty acids which are not manufactured by the body and are provided through diet and skin-care products, inhibiting the growth of some bacteria and protecting the skin against infection. They also have moisturizing properties. Essential fatty acids affect blood clotting, the transport of oxygen by the bloodstream to cells, tissues, and organs, lubrication and binding together of cells, and the availability of certain vitamins and minerals to the body. Oils which are especially good providers of essential fatty acids include: sunflower, safflower, evening primrose, borage, Rosa Mosqueta rosehip seed, kukui nut, and wheatgerm oils.

Essential Oil — see "Pure Essential Oil"

Extract — Often a concentrated form of plant material. Some plant material is not released completely by just a cold-pressing of the material; these plant materials are better extracted when passed through a solvent (can be organic or synthetic). Depending upon the desired state of the final product (powder, water-soluble liquid, or oil-soluble liquid), some solvents are removed after expression, and some are left as a part of the plant extract. Always ask for oil-soluble extracts, extracted without synthetic intrusion.

Fat — Primarily saturated (though not always) compounds of carbon, hydrogen, and oxygen that are attached to glycerol in the form of glycerides, obtained from animals and plants. They are normally, though not always, solid at room temperature, and they offer emollient properties.

Fatty acid — Saturated and unsaturated organic compounds of carbon, oxygen and hydrogen found in animal and vegetable fats and oils that occur naturally in the form of glycerides, a compound of glycerol and fatty acids, or what are called neutral oils. Fatty acids can be isolated from the glyceride through a process called hydrolysis. They must not be thought of as a burning acid, but rather as mild, emollient acids. Fatty acids are wonderful emollients.

Fragrance oil — A synthetic imitation of a pure essential oil. Fragrance oils do not offer the botanical properties found within pure essential oils and they often interfere with the saponification process.

Free-fatty acid — Those fatty acids which are not bonded to glycerol in the form of a triglyceride, but instead exist indepently in a "free" state. They are less stable than the complete triglyceride, and they contribute to rancidity.

Glyceride — A compound of alcohol plus an acid. Neutral oils contain glycerides of glycerol (the alcohol) plus a variety of fatty acids (the acid). When three molecules of fatty acid are attached to one molecule of glycerol,

the combination is known as a triglyceride.

Glycerin — A syrupy alcohol derived from vegetable oils and released from the glycerides during soapmaking. Although often removed as a by-product of the soap industry, cold-process soaps retain this natural glycerin and benefit from its emollient and humectant qualities. Glycerin is also known as glycerol and by the trade name, glycerine.

Grapefruit seed extract — This material extracted from grapefruit seeds is used as a natural preservative within soap. It should be added to the oil phase of the soapmaking process, as it will precipitate out of the lye solution.

Humectant — A substance which attracts and holds moisture to the skin; for example, a thin layer of either glycerin or aloe vera draws moisture from the air to soften the skin.

Hydrocarbon — Chemical compounds which contain only carbon and hydrogen atoms. Petroleum products are hydrocarbons. Much controversy surrounds this group of materials: some chemists consider petroleum products as natural, since they come from the earth and were once vegetation; opponents point to their altered state once synthetics are introduced in order to refine them for personal use. These products can be allergenic and phototoxic.

Hydrogenation — The process of adding hydrogen to the double bonds of unsaturated oils to solidify them and to make them more stable against oxidation and rancidity. Warning: any benefits must be weighed against the loss of essential fatty acids which are destroyed during the hydrogenation process.

Lye — Lye can be defined as either the solid caustic (such as sodium hydroxide) or as the liquid solution made by dissolving NaOH (in this case) beads or flakes into water.

Natural — A material which does not contain synthetic chemicals. Watch for products labeled "natural" which contain some organic substances, but also contain synthetic additives or preservatives.

Nutrient — An ingredient chosen for its beneficial properties. Within soapmaking, a nutrient is a material added to the formula for its ability to act upon the skin in a desired way.

Oil — Primarily unsaturated (though not always) compounds of carbon, hydrogen, and oxygen that are attached to glycerol in the form of glycerides, obtained from plants and animals. Oils are most often liquid at room temperature.

Organic — If a substance is organic, it is, or was at some point, alive and has not been altered with synthetic materials.

pH — When one hydrogen atom exists on its own, it is a positively charged hydrogen ion. The hydroxyl ion (OH — one oxygen atom and one hydrogen atom bonded together) is negatively charged and the balance of these hydrogen and hydroxyl ions within a solution dramatically affects the solution's makeup. An imbalance leaves the solution either acidic (more hydrogen ions) or alkaline (more hydroxyl ions). pH is a scale used to measure the hydrogen ion concentration of a substance.

At pH 7, the balance is just right. When there are more positive hydrogen ions, a material is acidic, somewhere between 1 and 7 on the pH scale. When there are more hydroxyl ions, the substance is alkaline or basic, somewhere between 7 and 14 on the pH scale.

Photosensitizers — Substances which make the skin sensitive and reactive to the sun's energy, especially light.

Potassium hydroxide — A strong, caustic base, also known as lye. Potassium hydroxide, or caustic potash, was the alkali used most throughout history to produce soap. Water steeped through wood ashes yields this caustic chemical which reacts with fats or oils to form liquid soaps and soft soaps.

Preservative — A substance used to slow down bacterial growth and decomposition. Look to natural preservatives for a one year shelf life; however, avoid synthetic preservatives which can offer years of shelf life, but adulterate a pure product.

Pure essential oil — The highly concentrated volatile oil obtained from plants which carry the scent and the beneficial properties of the particular plants. They are volatile because they evaporate quickly at room temperature when exposed to air. Watch for synthetic imitations which do not offer the botanical properties and which are less stable throughout the soapmaking process.

Rancidity — The decomposition of a substance which leads to a spoiled quality and odor.

Refinement — A process used to remove the impurities within a fat or an oil. Cold-pressed oils, those oils released without applying heat, contain the least amount of impurities and do not require refining — any impurities found within a cold-pressed oil can be filtered out. Pressing coarse meal further, while heating it, releases more oil, but this oil usually contains a higher percentage of non-glyceride impurities, like free fatty acids. Don't think of impurities so much as unclean, inferior materials, but rather as out of solution wanderers which are less stable and more likely to react because they are separate from the neutral oil. These are the culprits which can start reacting with the wrong mates, causing rancidity of the oil, and eventually our soaps. When an oil is refined, it is combined with an alkali solution, encouraging the non-glyceride portion to react with the alkali to form soap. The soap is drawn off, leaving the oil behind to be washed of any excess alkali or soap.

Rendering — The process of heating beef fat with water and salt, eventually leaving a clean, pure tallow which can be strained, cooled, and finally sliced away from the impurities.

Salt — Compounds that result from the replacement of part or all of the hydrogen of an acid by a metal. In soapmaking, sodium hydroxide replaces the hydrogen in the fatty acids (the fats or oils) to make a salt (or soap) of those fatty acids.

Saponification — The conversion of a fat or oil and an alkali into soap and glycerin.

Saponification value — This measures the amount of potassium hydroxide (in milligrams) required to saponify one gram of that particular

fat or oil. Also known as SAP value.

Setting up — As the soap mixture converts from a liquid to a solid state, the soap is "setting up." This process should take place in the frames, and not in the soap pan. Occasionally, a synthetic fragrance oil, or certain pure essential oils will cause the soap to begin setting up right in the soap pan, making it very difficult to pour the soap into the frames.

Sebum — A fatty substance secreted by the skin's sebaceous glands. Sebum lubricates the skin; however, without proper hygiene, the oil can build up and plug the pores, creating a breeding ground for bacterial growth, inflammation, and infection.

Soap — A mixture of salts of various fatty acids made by an alkali acting on the fatty acids. Fats or oils mixed with an alkali form soap and free glycerin; the resulting soap is a cleansing product.

Soda ash — Sodium carbonate, a grayish-white, powdery residue which forms on the surface of the soaps once they are exposed to air. Sodium hydroxide reacts with water or air to form this compound, which is not as harsh as sodium hydroxide, but is still drying to the skin. Slice 1/16 inch off of each bar to remove this substance.

Sodium hydroxide — A strong caustic base, also known as lye or caustic soda. This highly alkaline chemical can combine with fats or oils to form hard soaps.

Superfatting — To superfat a soap is to leave unsaponified oils in the final bars for a less harsh and more emollient soap. These unsaponified oils do not form compounds with the other soapmaking components, but instead remain in their original form within the bars. Superfatted soaps are more prone to rancidity, but worth the reduced shelf life.

Surfactant — A substance which reduces surface tension (the tight molecular bonds). For example, water molecules are tightly bonded, so water beads up on fabric, rather than soaking in to wet it. A surfactant, like soap, breaks down the bonds and enables it to spread and evenly wet the fabric.

Synergism — When two or more substances work together to create a benefit greater than the sum of each individual benefit.

Synthetic — A substance which is produced or altered artificially.

Tallow — The fat from the fatty tissue of cattle, sheep, and horses used for thousands of years to make soap. It may, however, cause eczema and blackheads.

Tocopherols — A classification in the vitamin E group. Fat-soluble, antioxidant compounds of vitamin E that are used to preserve soap. Look for the natural tocopherol made from vegetable sources and avoid the synthetic imitations. Note that tocopherols pro-

tect tallow and lard soaps better than they protect vegetable soaps.

Triglyceride — Fats and oils found in nature are almost always found in the form of triglycerides. These are different arrangements of fatty acids and glycerol (a form of glycerin): three (tri) fatty acids link to one molecule of glycerol to form a triglyceride, which will usually contain two or three different fatty acids, rather than just one kind of fatty acid.

Unsaponifiables — The portion of a neutral oil (including squalene, sterols, and fatty alcohols) which do not participate in the soapmaking reaction, but rather retain their original makeup in the final bars of soap.

Veganism — A philosophy based upon the belief that animals should not be killed or treated with cruelty, even for the benefit of mankind. In practice, this means eating no meat, fish, honey and dairy products, including butter, eggs and milk. Vegans (those who practice veganism) choose not to wear wool, leather, or fur, and they do not use any products which have been tested for safety on animals.

RELATED READING MATERIAL

Bramson, Ann Sela. *Soap: Making It, Enjoying It.* New York: Workman Publishing Company, 1975.

This is a wonderful book for the beginning soapmaker. It is readable, it offers step-by-step instruction for soapmaking, and it provides a few different recipes using easily accessible fats and oils. This book's weakness is the absence of a discussion of chemistry, including how to substitute one fat or oil for another. It also deals almost exclusively with tallow bars, offering just one vegetable soap recipe, without an explanation of how the vegetable soapmaking process differs from the tallow process. Nonetheless, this book pioneered the way for soapmakers who want to make their own soap and control what goes into the soap pan. This little paperback is inexpensive and worthwhile.

CTFA International Buyers' Guide 1993, The Cosmetic, Toiletry, and Fragrance Association, 1101 17th Street, NW, Suite 300, Washington, DC 20036-4702 202-331-1770

This is a carefully updated, well-organized trade journal listing materials and suppliers. The layout makes it cleaner reading than other journals which cram the writing on the page. Large, easy-to-read print.

Dadd, Debra Lynn. *Nontoxic, Natural, & Earthwise.* New York: The Putnam Publishing Group, 1990.

This book discusses the safety and the environmental impact of soaps, a variety of cosmetics, preservatives, colorants, fragrances, and virtually any product that comes to mind. Also included are comprehensive lists of non-toxic, natural, and earthwise products available through retail and mail order sources, though even just a few years later, the list is already somewhat outdated, with some of the suppliers out of business. Worthwhile reading.

DCI Directory Issue, Advanstar Communications, 207 Madison Ave., New York, NY 10016 218-723-9477

Good trade journal for soapmakers looking for a list of materials and their respective suppliers. Use in combination with other publications, since no one journal has a complete listing.

Ekiguchi, Kunio. *Gift Wrapping: Creative Ideas from Japan.* Tokyo: Kodansha International Ltd., 1985.

I spotted this book a couple of years ago and bought it with no intention to relate it to my soaps. At a quick glance, it seemed unusual and beautiful. A careful reading later revealed a treasure of ideas, from the materials themselves to the folding techniques. Each design is a work of art, doable by even the un-crafty. The ideas are inspiring and the instructions are easy to follow. One flip through this book inspires us to put time and thought into presentation, and to not ignore this final touch. This is simple elegance.

Hampton, Aubrey. **Natural Organic Hair and Skin Care.** Tampa, Florida: Organica Press, 1987.

A tremendous volume of research, sometimes overwhelming as it reads like a textbook, but definitely worth the time and concentration required to read thoroughly. This book leaves the careful reader with a real knowledge of how the skin works and therefore which materials are helpful or harmful. This is one of the most compelling and scholarly discussions of natural versus synthetic skin-care products and their preservatives. The soapmaker will be disappointed by the absence of a chapter on soaps, but not one chapter in this book is irrelevant to the soapmaker. An understanding of the skin and how it incorporates a variety of materials will make us all better soapmakers.

Kirk, R.E. and D.F. Othmer. **Kirk Othmer Encyclopedia of Chemical Technology,** 3rd Ed. New York: John Wiley & Sons.

This encyclopedia is the most comprehensive set available, readable for the chemistry student, and detailed enough for the chemist. Arranged alphabetically in volumes, the soapmaker can research all facets of the chemistry of soapmaking.

J. Davidsohn, E.J., and Better, A. Davidsohn. **Soap Manufacture,** Volume I. New York: Interscience Publishers, Inc., 1953.

This is a standard old volume. It is very helpful to the soapmaker who

wants to understand more about the chemistry of soapmaking and the various methods used over the years within industry to manufacture soap. The cold-process soapmaker looking only for practical tips will have to sift through pages and pages of technical information to find a relevant tidbit here and there. Also, the couple of pages written on the cold-process are outdated, as we now use refined vegetable oils more and more often than the tallow/coconut combination of yesteryear. We therefore use different techniques and temperatures than this book describes. Note that this volume often refers the reader to Volumes II and III for even more information on soapmaking, but these volumes were never written.

Journal of the American Oil Chemists' Society. Champagne, Illinois: American Oil Chemists' Society.

This journal is a set of articles, arranged alphabetically by subject, and bound into volumes. One volume, devoted solely to index, leads the reader to all relevant articles. This is highly technical, relating only to fats and oils. Universities and larger libraries will have this set in their science departments.

Larabre, Marcel. **Aromatherapy Workbook.** Rochester, VT: Healing Arts Press, 1990.

So many of the aromatherapy books simply list plants and describe the benefits of the many essential oils. They often include a history of aromatherapy and some recipes. In favorable contrast, The Aromatherapy

Workbook stands out as a comprehensive work, offering a full discussion of the oils, the extraction processes, the principles of blending, and synthetic oils versus natural oils. It skillfully explains the chemistry of essential oils.

Milwidsky, B. *Soap and Detergent Technology,* reprinted from Household & Personal Products Industry (HAPPI). Ramsey, NJ: Rodham Publishing, 1980.

This magazine is reprinted from HAPPI, and, though it more often discusses soapmaking within the industrial setting, this particular issue contains a section on oils, fats and fatty acids, and a section on saponification. Though it, too, is written to industry, the cold-process soapmaker can pick up some basic soapmaking chemistry without having to read through hundreds of pages of technical writing. Written more as a long article and not a book, this work can only go into just so much detail and depth. But for a good, solid overview with enough detail to educate, this well written article starts at the beginning and does a good job explaining the chemistry of soapmaking.

Mohr, Merilyn. *The Art of Soapmaking.* Ontario, Canada: Camden House Publishing, 1988.

This book is well written, and it, like Ann Bramson's book, offers the beginning soapmaker a very readable manual. But *The Art of Soapmaking* is stronger in its text and research than it is with respect to its formulations. It offers a nice variety of recipes, incorporating all kinds of nutrients, but I had trouble with many of the recipes. The soapmaking instruction section is too general for the soapmaker desperate for step-by-step detail, and the recipes are measured by volume rather than weight, a less precise method. Do read this book to pick up ideas, but do not rely upon these recipes exclusively for calculations.

Spitz, Luis. *Soap Technology For The 1990's.* Champagne, Illinois: American Oil Chemists' Society, 1990.

Within this volume, a few different authors present different facets of the soapmaking industry. Chapters One and Two explain the history of soapmaking and the chemistry of soapmaking with enough detail to be quite useful. But the remainder of this expensive book seems to be written for industrial soap manufacturers. *Soap Technology For The 1990's* does just that: it discusses the processing, formulation, and packaging of modern industrial soapmaking, including a discussion of synthetic soaps and the particular bar soaps sold on the market today. None of the book offers practical advice for the cold-process soapmaker.

Stanislaus, Ignatius Valerius Stanley. *American Soap Maker's Guide.* New York: Henry Carey Baird & Co., Inc., 1928.

More like the very old treatises on soapmaking, this book deals primarily with making soaps industrially. However, in combination with more updated material, this work is valuable even to the cold-process soapmaker. Like

Soap Manufacture, it does a nice job discussing soapmaking materials and the science of the process.

Swern, Daniel. *Bailey's Industrial Oil and Fat Products. Vol. 1,* 4th Ed. New York: John Wiley & Sons, 1979.

Though costly, this book offers enough usable information to make it worth the expense for the soapmaker who wants much more than an overview. The first half of this volume is devoted wholly to the structure and composition of fats and oils, discussing fatty acids in great detail. The chapter on soapmaking toward the end of the book is weak, and it deals only with the manufacture of soaps within industry. Look to other material for soapmaking instructions, and use this only as a reference book. Be warned that this volume is highly technical, and should only be purchased by someone looking for great detail about the chemical makeup of fats, oils, and fatty acids.

The Business of Herbs. Northwind Farm Publications, RR2 Box 246, Shevlin, MN 56676-9535.

This is a bimonthly trade magazine, a news and resource journal for herb businesses. Occasionally relevant to the soapmaker, but always helpful to herb-related cottage industries. Includes updates on technology, marketing ideas, retail trends, book reviews, conference listings, and resource guides.

The Herb Companion. Interweave Press, 201 East Fourth Street, Loveland, CO 80537 (800) 272-2193.

My favorite pleasure magazine. Only a few years old, the Herb Companion has matured into a full-scale publication. The articles are well written and meaty, detailing the many uses of herbs. The gardener, the herbalist, the artisan, and the soapmaker often share an interest in botanicals, untainted products, and environmental issues. We are all interested in one another and the ties which bind, and this magazine pulls us all together. Keep this magazine in mind as a good spot to advertise your natural soaps.

In the same series:

The Herbal Body Book: A Natural Approach to Healthier Hair, Skin, and Nails by Stephanie Tourles
Over 100 recipes to make facial scrubs, hair rinses, shampoos, cleansing lotions, lip balms, powders, insect repellants, and more from common herbs, fruits, and grains. 128 pages.

Other herb-related topics:

A Gift Book of Herbs and Herbal Flowers edited by Rosemary Hemphill
Includes a potpourri of herb and flower prose, poems, recipes, crafts, and folklore. Full-color botanical drawings, watercolors, and contemporary photographs featuring 32 herbs and flowers. 112 pages.

At Home with Herbs: Inspiring Ideas for Cooking, Crafts, Decorating and Cosmetics by Jane Newdick
Over 1000 herbal projects for crafters, home decorators, chefs, and naturalists. Includes information on planting, harvesting, and storing herbs. 224 pages.

Growing & Using Herbs Successfully by Betty E.M. Jacobs
Guide to planting, propagating, harvesting, drying, freezing, and storing 64 popular herbs. 240 pages.

Growing Your Herb Business by Bertha Reppert
Practical advice on every aspect of starting and maintaining an herb business, including developing products, packaging, special events, mail order, newsletters, and business procedures. From the founder of *The Rosemary House*. 192 pages.

The Herbal Tea Garden: Planning, Planting, Harvesting & Brewing by Marietta Marshall Marcin
Complete handbook for herbal tea lovers who want to select, grow, and create their own special brews from 70 herbal tea plants. 224 pages.

Herbal Treasures: Inspiring Month-by-Month Projects for Gardening, Cooking, and Crafts by Phyllis V. Shaudys
A compendium of the best herb crafts, recipes, and gardening ideas from herb experts across the country. 320 pages.

Herbal Vinegar by Maggie Oster
Instructions for making inexpensive and easy herb, spice, vegetable, and flower vinegars, along with more than 100 recipes for using them in everything from appetizers, soups, and salsas, to entrees. 176 pages.

The Pleasure of Herbs: A Month-by-Month Guide to Growing, Using, and Enjoying Herbs by Phyllis Shaudys
Packed full of information about herbs and herb growing, with indoor and outdoor herb-growing directions, recipes, and craft projects for every month of the year. 288 pages.

These books are available at your bookstore, lawn and garden center, or directly from Storey Publishing, Department WM, Schoolhouse Road, Pownal, Vermont 05261. To order toll-free by phone, call 1-800-441-5700.

INDEX

Maine, Sandy, 146–47, 165
Maple Hill Farm, 141, 165
Measuring, note about, 80
Milled soap
    colorants in, 53
    hand-cut versus, 13–14
Mineral pigments, 53, 56
Mixed Nuts Bar, 123
Mixture, diagnosing problems
        with, 127–28
Mizuhiki cord, 140, 161
Molding, decorative, 133–34
Molecular weights of fatty acids,
    151
Montmorillonite, 160

N

*Natural Organic Hair and Skin
    Care* (Hampton), 72, 131
Natural soap, synthetic versus, 16
Nature's Acres, 69, 165
Nutrients
    See also under type of
    defined, 58

O

Oatmeal/honey, as a nutrient,
    66–67
Oatmeal/Honey Soap, 122
Oils
    See also under type of
    cost and availability of, 8
    fatty-acid makeup of, 150
    iodine value of, 152
    mixing fats and, 149–50
    SAP chart for, 153
    suppliers for, 158–61
Oleic acid, 28, 148
Olein, 148
Olive oil
    caution when using, 22
    characteristics of, 22–24
    cost and availability of, 8,

22–23
    fatty-acid makeup of, 150
    grades of, 22–23
    lather ability of, 11, 24
    moisture absorption and, 11
    pomace, 22, 23
    suppliers of, 160
One-Stop Soap, 102–6

P

Palm Christi oil. *See* Castor oil
Palm kernel oil
    characteristics of, 25, 27
    cost and availability of, 27
    lather ability of, 27
    suppliers of, 160
Palm oil
    characteristics of, 24–25
    cost and availability of, 8,
        24–25
    fatty-acid makeup of, 150
    lather ability of, 25
    suppliers of, 160
Peanut oil
    characteristics of, 27–28
    cost and availability of, 8, 27
    lather ability of, 11
    suppliers of, 160
Pearlescent pigments, 56–57
pH, testing for, 127, 131
Plant oils and extracts
    as colorants, 55
    suppliers of, 160
Potassium hydroxide, 31
Preservatives
    carrot root oil, 74–75
    defined, 70
    grapefruit seed extract, 73–74
    natural, 71–72
    selecting, 72–73
    synthetic, to avoid, 70
    tocopherols, 74
Problems, diagnosing, 127–31